Case Studies for the Medical Office

Capstone Billing Simulation

Fifth Edition

Susan M. Sanderson

 Higher Education

Boston   Burr Ridge, IL   Dubuque, IA   New York   San Francisco   St. Louis
Bangkok   Bogotá   Caracas   Kuala Lumpur   Lisbon   London   Madrid   Mexico City
Milan   Montreal   New Delhi   Santiago   Seoul   Singapore   Sydney   Taipei   Toronto

Mc Graw Hill Higher Education

CASE STUDIES FOR THE MEDICAL OFFICE: CAPSTONE BILLING SIMULATION

Published by McGraw-Hill, a business unit of The McGraw-Hill Companies, Inc., 1221 Avenue of the Americas, New York, NY, 10020. Copyright © 2010 by The McGraw-Hill Companies, Inc. All rights reserved. Previous editions © 1999, 2003, 2005, and 2007. No part of this publication may be reproduced or distributed in any form or by any means, or stored in a database or retrieval system, without the prior written consent of The McGraw-Hill Companies, Inc., including, but not limited to, in any network or other electronic storage or transmission, or broadcast for distance learning.

Some ancillaries, including electronic and print components, may not be available to customers outside the United States.

✪ This book is printed on acid-free paper.

3 4 5 6 7 8 9 0 QPD/QPD 0

ISBN 978-0-07-340200-0
MHID 0-07-340200-1

Vice president/Editor in chief: *Elizabeth Haefele*
Vice president/Director of marketing: *John E. Biernat*
Sponsoring editor: *Natalie J. Ruffatto*
Director of development, Allied Health: *Patricia Hesse*
Developmental editor: *Bonnie Hemrick*
Executive marketing manager: *Roxan Kinsey*
Lead media producer: *Damian Moshak*
Media producer: *Marc Mattson*
Director, Editing/Design/Production: *Jess Ann Kosic*
Lead project manager: *Rick Hecker*

Senior production supervisor: *Janean A. Utley*
Designer: *Marianna Kinigakis*
Media project manager: *Mark A. S. Dierker*
Outside development house: *Susan Magovern, Chestnut Hill*
Cover design: *Jessica M. Lazar*
Typeface: *12/16 Minion*
Compositor: *Aptara, Inc.*
Printer: *Quebecor World Dubuque Inc.*
Cover credit: © Gunay Mutlu/Stockphoto

Codeveloped by McGraw-Hill Higher Education and Chestnut Hill Enterprises, Inc. chestnuthl@aol.com

The Medisoft Student Data files, illustrations, instructions, and exercises in *Case Studies for the Medical Office: Capstone Billing Simulation* are compatible with the Medisoft™ Advanced Version 14 Patient Accounting software available at the time of publication. Adaptations may be necessary for use with subsequent versions of the software. Text changes will be made in reprints when possible. Medisoft Advanced Version 14 software must be available to access the Medisoft Student Data files. It can be obtained by contacting your McGraw-Hill sales representative.

All brand or product names are trademarks or registered trademarks of their respective companies.

CPT five-digit codes, nomenclature, and other data are copyright 2008 American Medical Association. All rights reserved. No fee schedules, basic unit, relative values, or related listings are included in the CPT. The AMA assume no liability for the data contained herein.

CPT codes are based on CPT 2009.
ICD-9-CM codes are based on ICD-9-CM 2009.

All names, situations, and anecdotes are fictitious. They do not represent any person, event, or medical record.

Library of Congress Cataloging-in-Publication Data

Sanderson, Susan M.
   Case studies for the medical office : Capstone billing simulation / Susan M. Sanderson. — 5th ed.
      p. ; cm.
   Includes index.
   ISBN-13: 978-0-07-340200-0 (alk. paper)
   ISBN-10: 0-07-340200-1 (alk. paper)
   1. Medical assistants—Case studies. 2. Medical offices—Case studies. 3. Medical fees—Computer programs—Case studies. I. Title.
   [DNLM: 1. Fees and Charges—Problems and Exercises. 2. Forms and Records Control—Problems and Exercises. 3. Office Automation—Problems and Exercises. 4. Practice Management—economics—Problems and Exercises. 5. Reimbursement Mechanisms—Problems and Exercises. 6. Software—Problems and Exercises. W 18.2 S216ca 2010]
   R728.8.S258 2010
   651'.9610285—dc22

                                    2008050308

The Internet addresses listed in the text were accurate at the time of publication. The inclusion of a Web site does not indicate an endorsement by the authors or McGraw-Hill, and McGraw-Hill does not guarantee the accuracy of the information presented at these sites.

www.mhhe.com

Table of Contents

■■■ PART 3

On the Job 85

▬ PART 4

Source Documents   165

Preface

Case Studies for the Medical Office provides students with enhanced learning opportunities that lead to superior qualifications for employment in medical offices. The text/workbook contains a realistic and extensive simulation covering two weeks of billing work in a medical office. Students use Medisoft Advanced Patient Accounting, a widely distributed medical office administrative software program, to complete the simulation. In addition to practicing and reinforcing their Medisoft skills, *Case Studies for the Medical Office* introduces fourteen new Medisoft training topics that expand their knowledge. Students must exhibit critical thinking and problem solving to pull together the resources they will need to handle their daily assignments.

The program builds important skills for handling computerized billing tasks in medical offices. While performing various jobs during the simulation, students reinforce essential skills such as inputting patient information, scheduling appointments, and handling billing, reports, and insurance claims. In addition, students must exhibit the ability to research facts, think through priorities, and analyze problems. All these skills and competencies are readily transferred from *Case Studies for the Medical Office* to billing positions in medical offices, regardless of the particular billing software in use.

The prerequisite for successful completion of *Case Studies for the Medical Office* is a basic knowledge of Medisoft Advanced, which can be gained by studying McGraw-Hill publications such as *Computers in the Medical Office* or *Patient Billing*. An understanding of the concepts and procedures for medical coding, billing, and reimbursement is also very helpful. This background can be obtained by studying McGraw-Hill's related insurance titles, the briefer, focused *From Patient to Payment* (Newby) or the longer, comprehensive *Medical Insurance* (Valerius/Bayes/Newby/Seggern).

Computer Supplies and Equipment

The Medisoft Student Data files, available at the book's website (www.mhhe.com/casestudies5e), provide a database of case study information. Other equipment and supplies needed are as follows:

- PC with 500 MHz or greater processor speed
- 256 MB RAM
- 500 MB available hard disk space (if saving data to hard disk)
- CD-ROM 2x or faster disk drive

- Windows Vista Business 32-bit version (Medisoft 14 will not work on the 64-bit system), Windows XP Professional, or Windows 2000 Professional
- Medisoft™ Advanced Version 14 Patient Accounting software
- External storage device for storing backup copies of the working database
- Printer
- Active Internet connection to access the book's website

Medisoft™ Advanced Version 14 Patient Accounting software is available to schools adopting *Case Studies for the Medical Office*. Please contact your McGraw-Hill sales representative for information about receiving the software. Information on ordering and installing the software is also located at the book's website, www.mhhe.com/casestudies5e. Student-at-Home Software Medisoft Advanced Version 14 is available as an option for distance education or for students who want to practice with the software at home.

Supplementary Material

The online Instructor's Manual provides the instructor with a course overview, information on ordering and installing Medisoft Advanced software, lesson plans and teaching suggestions, a pretest covering basic Medisoft knowledge, and answer keys for the simulation exercises. Three correlation tables are also included: SCANS, AAMA Role Delineation Study Areas of Competence (2003), and AMT Registered Medical Assistant Certification Exam Topics.

In addition, the instructor section of the book's website contains the following supplementary materials: a PowerPoint slide presentation, answers to Part 1 and Part 2 Quizzes, answers to Part 3 Daily Worksheets, Troubleshooting Tips, and a series of backup files for Part 3 to help teachers evaluate students' work at the end of each day and week. By restoring the backup file for a given day, the instructor has easy access to the current state of the database when the exercises for that chapter have been completed.

Acknowledgments

We are grateful to the following individuals for their insightful reviews, criticisms, and helpful suggestions.

Fifth Edition Reviewers:

Patricia Casey, MBE
Trident Technical College

Carol Hinricher
University of Montana College of Technology

Patricia Jarvis
Truckee Meadows Community College

Krista Mahan, MA
Walla Walla Community College

Revel Metzger, MA, AA
Elizabethtown Community and Technical College

Susan Scalzi, BS, CBCS
Delaware County Community College

Robin Smith, CMA, CBCS, RHE
Macomb Community College

Carole A. Zeglin, MS, BS, RMA
Westmoreland County Community College

Susan D. Steinriede, EdD
Trident Technical College

Cynthia Zumbrun, MEd, RHIT, CCS-P
Allegany College of Maryland

Nancy Thiele, BS, AA
Truckee Meadows Community College

Stacey Wilson, MHA, MT/PBT(ASCP), CMA
Program Coordinator,
Cabarrus College of Health Sciences

Symposium Attendees:

Kelli Batten
Career Technical College

Samantha Lopez
Career Point Institute

Kelley Fazzone
Blair College

Wilsetta McClain
Dorsey Schools

Stephanie Hales
Parks College

Cari McPherson
Ross Medical Education Center

Gladys Hammic
McLennan Community College

Elaine Miyamoto
Robert Morris College

Denise Harris
Georgia Medical Institute

Angela Parmley
Sanford Brown Institute

Lucinda Ionno
Stark State College of Technology

Lilia Torres
Florida Career College

Amy Lee
Valencia Community College

Yolando Savoy
Medical Career Institute

Previous Edition Reviewers:

Marcia Banks
Chubb University

Lynn Harris
Baker College

Russell Battiata
Medvance College

Toni Hartley
3 Powerhouse Road

Jonathan Dockery
Maric-Carson

Lisa Hauschild
Ivy Tech State College

Yolande Gardner
Bessemer State Tech College

Tim McDonald
Southern Maine College

Sandy Minnick
Business Institute of PA

Mary Jane Montgomery
ETI Tech College

Nancy Moorehead
Eastern New Mexico University

Debora Mullen
Sanford Brown Institute

Tomma Parco
Pueblo Community College

Michelle Sechrist
ATI Career Center Training

Geiselle Thompson
Quality Staffing Agency

Jim Wallace
Maric-Los Angeles

Kim Wallace Foster
NW Business College

Stacey Wilson
Cabarrus College

Getting Started

Case Studies for the Medical Office has four parts. This section describes each part and explains how each part is used in the text/workbook. It also provides information on downloading the Medisoft Student Data files that are used in the simulation exercises, as well as instructions on backing up and restoring files in Medisoft.

Part 1

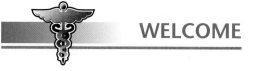

Part 1, *Introduction to Polaris Medical Group,* sets the stage for the rest of the text/workbook. Part 1 is based on the premise that Polaris Medical Group (PMG) has recently hired you. PMG is a general practice with a complex environment of patient cases, insurance affiliations, and schedule demands. Part 1 introduces the practice's staff, describes the guidelines for working with medical office records, and details the role of the patient services specialist, which you will perform in the simulation. An objective quiz at the end of this part is intended to test your comprehension of this introductory material.

Part 2

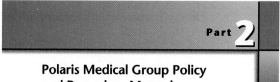

Part 2, *Polaris Medical Group Policy and Procedure Manual,* covers the practice's general policies and employment procedures. Part 2 has detailed guidelines on processing new patient registration and referrals, scheduling appointments, and billing. It also contains detailed information sheets on the insurance carriers with which the practice interacts. An objective quiz at the end of Part 2 will help you assess your grasp of the key points.

Part 3

Part 3, *On the Job,* requires you to perform a series of assignments using Medisoft Advanced Patient Accounting. Each day of the ten-day assignment at Polaris Medical Group contains applications of the knowledge required in a medical office. Medisoft training topics are introduced in the text at the points you need the knowledge to complete the specific tasks.

To assist you, special tips are provided in Part 3. You will also need to refer to the Health Plan Information Pages at the end of Part 2 for details about the insurance coverage percentages for the health plans used in Part 3. At the end of each day's jobs in Part 3, a Daily Worksheet is provided to help verify that your work was completed correctly.

Part 4

Part 4, *Source Documents,* provides the patient data needed to complete the daily tasks in Part 3. The variety of completed forms, similar to those used in medical offices, includes patient information forms, encounter forms, physician's notes, chart notes, remittance advices, and audit/edit reports.

When you complete the assignments in *Case Studies for the Medical Office,* you will be well prepared to handle a billing position in a medical office. Even if you do not use Medisoft on the job, the skills you practice here will be similar to those skills needed to use almost any medical accounting program.

Using Medisoft

Before a medical office begins to use Medisoft, basic information about the practice and its patients must be entered in the program. This preliminary work has been done for you. The medical practice with which you will work is called Polaris Medical Group (PMG). Check with your instructor to determine whether the Medisoft Student Data files, which contain the PMG database, have already been loaded on your computer.

If your instructor has not already loaded the files, go to the book's website at www.mhhe. com/casestudies5e to download them at this time. You will need to load the Medisoft Student Data files before you start the jobs in Part 3.

Backing Up Data in Medisoft

Many practices back up data at the end of each day. A copy of backup data is usually stored at a location other than the office, in case of a natural or man-made disaster at the office facility. In a school setting, files are also backed up regularly to store each student's work securely and separately.

If you are in a school environment, it is important to make a backup copy of your work after each Medisoft session. This ensures that you can restore your work during the next session and be able to use your own data even if another student uses the computer after you or if, for any reason, the files on the school computer are changed or corrupted. This section provides instructions on backing up data in Medisoft.

1. You can use the Backup option on the File menu to back up your data at any time. However, by default, Medisoft also gives you the opportunity to back up your data each time you exit the program. Click the Exit option on the File menu to exit Medisoft.

2. The Backup Reminder dialog box appears. You will back up your data to the folder on your hard drive where you stored the original backup file, *polaris.mbk,* only you will back it up under a new name according to the day of the simulation you are working on in the text. Click the Back Up Data Now button.

3. The Backup dialog box appears. The Destination File Path and Name box at the top should already show the name of the folder on your hard drive where polaris.mbk is stored (whichever file was last used is displayed by default). If it does not show this path, use the Find button to locate this folder on your hard drive.

4. To back up the data under a new name, change the file name *polaris.mbk* at the end of the path name to ***Week1Day1.mbk*** (for the first day of the simulation). (*Hint:* Use the End key or the right arrow key on your keyboard to move the cursor to the end of the filename. Backspace over the old name, polaris.mbk, to erase it, and then key Week1Day1.mbk. You many want to add your initials to the beginning of the filename if you are sharing a drive.) Then click the Start Backup button.

5. Medisoft backs up the data under the new name and displays an Information box indicating that the backup is complete.

6. Click the OK button to close the Information dialog box and exit the Medisoft program.

7. For safekeeping, copy your new backup file from your hard drive to an external storage device, such as a flash drive or a CD-ROM. A separate backup copy prevents you from losing your work if the hard drive fails or if you or someone else accidentally deletes data on the computer.

Restoring Data in Medisoft

If you are sharing a computer with other students in a school environment, you will need to perform a restore before a new Medisoft session to be certain you are working with your own data. If necessary, follow these steps to restore your latest backup file.

To restore the file *Week1Day1.mbk* to C:\MediData\Polaris:

1. Copy your backup file from your external storage device to the assigned location on your hard drive. (Ask your instructor if you are not sure which folder this is.)

2. Start Medisoft.

3. Check the program's title bar at the top of the screen to make sure Polaris Medical Group is displayed as the active data set. (If it is not, use the Open Practice option on the File menu to select it.)

4. Open the File menu, and click Restore Data.

5. When the Warning box appears, click OK. The Restore dialog box appears.

6. Use the Find button to locate your assigned storage folder on the hard drive (the folder used in step 1 above). Locate *Week1Day1.mbk* in the list of existing backup

files displayed for that folder, and click on it to attach it to the Backup File Path and Name at the top of the dialog box. (The end of the path name should read \ . . . \ Week1Day1.mbk.)

7. The Destination Path at the bottom of the box should already be C:\MediData\Polaris.

8. Click the Start Restore button.

9. When the Confirm box appears, click OK.

10. An Information dialog box appears indicating that the restore is complete. You have successfully restored the *Week1Day1.mbk* file for use with Medisoft for the next session. Click OK to continue.

11. The Restore dialog box disappears. You are ready to begin working.

Introduction to Polaris Medical Group

LEARNING OUTCOMES

After successfully completing Part 1, you will be able to define the key terms and:

1.1 Describe the organization and staff of Polaris Medical Group.

1.2 List the types of information located in medical records.

1.3 Discuss the importance of confidentiality and patient privacy in the medical office.

1.4 Identify the general responsibilities of Polaris Medical Group employees.

1.5 Discuss the qualities and attitudes of an effective patient services specialist.

1.6 Identify the specific tasks that a patient services specialist at Polaris Medical Group performs during a typical day.

KEY TERMS

audit trail

documentation

electronic health record (EHR)

family practitioner

Health Insurance Portability and Accountability Act of 1996 (HIPAA)

HIPAA Electronic Health Care Transactions and Code Sets (TCS)

HIPAA Privacy Rule

HIPAA Security Rule

internist

medical record

National Provider Identifier (NPI)

primary care physician

protected health information (PHI)

SOAP format

This section is your introduction to Polaris Medical Group. You will learn about the purpose, the people, and the structure of the practice. In addition, you will be introduced to the topics of medical records and patient privacy. All staff members at Polaris Medical Group must understand the proper use and disclosure of patient health information.

Part 1 also provides information about the types of tasks you will complete in Part 3, On the Job. You will learn about your role and your specific responsibilities at Polaris Medical Group, including activities such as scheduling, billing, and responding to patient inquiries.

WELCOME

The physicians and staff of Polaris Medical Group (PMG) welcome you as a new member of our health care team. We are committed to providing each of our patients with the highest quality of health care. We hired you because we are confident that you can contribute to that goal. We are also committed to creating and maintaining a positive work environment for our employees.

At PMG, we work as a patient services team. The physicians, assistants, and medical office staff members work together, sharing information and resources to accomplish our common goals. We treat all patients and staff members with courtesy and patience. The caring environment we create is one reason that patients return to the clinic. A caring environment also makes the workplace a pleasant one for staff members. At PMG, we believe in treating others as we would like to be treated.

Statement of Purpose

Polaris Medical Group provides medical care and services to individuals and families regardless of age, race, color, creed, national origin, gender, or disability. As a family practice, we respond to a broad range of patient needs. Our primary function is to treat illness, disease, injury, and disability through evaluation, examination, and the use of medical procedures. We also educate individuals and families regarding preventive care. Our goal is to help all patients achieve their maximum potential within their capabilities and to accelerate convalescence and reduce the length of the patient's recovery.

Organization and Staff

family practitioner
a physician who treats patients of all ages and does not specialize in one area of medicine

internist a physician who specializes in the care of adults

The organization chart for PMG is illustrated in Figure 1-1. There are two physicians in the practice: Robin C. Crebore, M.D., F.A.A.F.P. (Fellow, American Academy of Family Physicians), and Michael P. Mahabir, M.D., F.A.C.P. (Fellow, American College of Physicians). Dr. Crebore, a *family practitioner*, has a general practice and treats patients of all ages. Dr. Mahabir, as an *internist*, specializes in the care of adults.

The physicians' backgrounds are as follows:

Robin C. Crebore, M.D., F.A.A.F.P.
Specialty: Family Practice
University: Fairfield University, CT
Medical School: Tufts University School of Medicine, MA, 1988
Internship: Presbyterian University of Pennsylvania Medical Center, 1989
Residency: St. Elizabeth's Hospital, MA, 1991

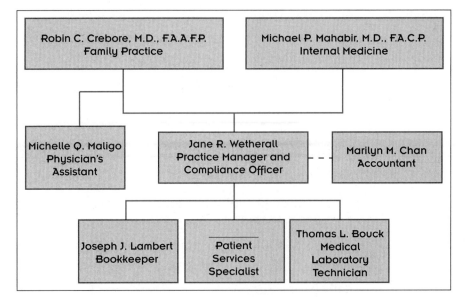

FIGURE 1-1 Organization Chart of Polaris Medical Group

Board Certification Date:

 1991, Family Practice

 1997, Recertified Family Practice

 1998, Certificate of Added Qualifications in Geriatrics

Memberships: Fellow, American Academy of Family Practitioners; American Geriatrics Society

Michael P. Mahabir, M.D., F.A.C.P.

Specialty: Internal Medicine

University: University of Colorado

Medical School: East Virginia Medical School, VA, 1994

Internship: Medical Center Hospital of Vermont, 1995

Residency: Medical Center Hospital of Vermont, 1997

Board Certification Date: 1997, Internal Medicine

Memberships: American Society of Internal Medicine; Fellow, American College of Physicians; Diplomat, American Board of Internal Medicine

Both physicians offer consultations for private patients, and they accept assignment for Medicare and Medicaid. Both are also identified as ***primary care physicians*** in a number of managed care plans. In this role, they are responsible for overseeing patients' overall health care and for referring their patients to specialists, such as cardiologists for cardiovascular disease or dermatologists for skin disease. Michelle Maligo, the office's physician's assistant, works with both physicians.

Jane Wetherall, our practice manager and compliance officer, is responsible for oversight of the medical office. You, the patient services specialist (PSS), report to her, as does Thomas Bouck, the part-time medical laboratory

primary care physician a physician in a managed care plan who directs all aspects of a patient's care, including routine services, referrals to specialists, and supervision of hospital admission technician. Accounting functions are handled by a bookkeeper, Joseph Lambert, whose work is checked by Marilyn Chan, an outside accountant who reviews the financial aspects of the practice.

Polaris Medical Group is located in a modern medical office building in Columbus, Ohio, three blocks from St. Mary's Hospital. Our offices have a patient reception area and a front office where the business transactions of the medical practice take place. Your desk is located in a glassed-in section of the front office. There is also a separate lunchroom.

Each doctor has a separate office. In addition, there are three examining rooms for the evaluation and treatment of patients and an office laboratory for analyzing blood and urine samples. PMG also contracts with an outside laboratory for other types of lab work. Specimens are picked up from the practice and processed on a daily basis.

MEDICAL RECORDS

medical record a file that includes the patient information form, the patient's medical history, record of care, progress notes, insurance correspondence, and other pertinent documents

electronic health record (EHR) patient medical record created using a computer

Patients' records are a critical component of all services and treatments we provide at PMG. *Medical records* contain all information pertaining to a patient's health history. They also contain all communications with and about each patient. The medical record begins with a patient's first contact with the practice and continues through all treatments and services. These records provide continuity and communication among physicians and other health care professionals who are involved in a patient's care.

In our practice, patient medical records are created on computers, rather than written by hand. In addition to physicians' notes, a patient's *electronic health record (EHR)* includes digital files of X-ray images, lab test results, medical history, and a picture of the patient. Electronic health records offer significant advantages over paper records. For example, a patient who is away from home or in an accident can authorize a local physician to access the record to locate needed history. In addition, large amounts of information gathered over many years about a patient's chronic condition can be organized for quick review.

Information in the Medical Record

documentation the recording of facts and observations about a patient's health status in a logical, chronological sequence

Information recorded in the patient's medical record is known as *documentation*. Accurate, complete documentation provides the physician with a detailed summary of each of the patient's visits, including information about treatments, progress, and outcomes.

The medical record originates when a patient visits the office for the first time. Using the information on the patient information form (see Figure 1-2), a patient

PATIENT INFORMATION FORM

THIS SECTION REFERS TO PATIENT ONLY

Name:	Sex:	Marital Status: ☐ S ☐ M ☐ D ☐ W	Birth Date:

Address:	SS#:

City: State: Zip:	Employer: Phone:

Home Phone:	Employer's Address:

Work Phone:	City: State: Zip:

Spouse's Name:	Spouse's Employer:

Emergency Contact:	Relationship: Phone #:

FILL IN IF PATIENT IS A MINOR

Parent/Guardian's Name:	Sex:	Marital Status: ☐ S ☐ M ☐ D ☐ W	Birth Date:

Phone:	SS#:

Address:	Employer: Phone:

City: State: Zip:	Employer's Address:

Student Status:	City: State: Zip:

INSURANCE INFORMATION

Primary Insurance Company:	Secondary Insurance Company:

Subscriber's Name: Birth Date:	Subscriber's Name: Birth Date:

Plan: SS#:	Plan:

Policy #: Group #:	Policy #: Group #:

Copayment/Deductible: Price Code:	

OTHER INFORMATION

Reason for visit:	Allergy to Medication (list):

Name of referring physician:	If auto accident, list date and state in which it occurred:

I authorize treatment and agree to pay all fees and charges for the person named above. I agree to pay all charges shown by statements, promptly upon their presentation, unless credit arrangements are agreed upon in writing.

I authorize payment directly to POLARIS MEDICAL GROUP of insurance benefits otherwise payable to me. I hereby authorize the release of any medical information necessary in order to process a claim for payment in my behalf.

_____   _____
(Patient's Signature/Parent or Guardian's Signature)   (Date)

I plan to make payment of my medical expenses as follows (check one or more):

_____ Insurance (as above)   _____ Cash/Check/Credit/Debit Card   _____ Medicare   _____ Medicaid   _____ Workers' Comp.

FIGURE 1-2 Patient Information Form

chart is created. After that, the medical record is updated each time the patient visits the physician. PMG includes the following items in every medical record:

- The patient's full name, Social Security number, date of birth, insurance information, and chart number
- A demographic page that lists the patient's complete address and phone number; occupation; name, address, and phone number of employer; and marital status
- The day, month, and year of each illness or injury
- A list of the patient's medical conditions, created and updated as needed

- A list of the patient's known allergies, created and updated as needed
- A list of all medications the patient is taking, created and updated as needed
- Immunization records
- Complete documentation for each new medical condition noted, including the relevant history, examination, assessment (diagnosis), treatment plan, outcome, and follow-up
- The patient's medical history, including illnesses, accidents, and surgeries
- Documentation of history regarding tobacco, alcohol, or substance abuse
- Results from laboratory, X-ray, or other medical tests, and physician's notes regarding the test results
- Photocopies of all prescriptions written for the patient
- Notes regarding phone calls with the patient or legal guardian, or phone calls to another physician about the patient's condition
- Any requests for information about the patient (from a health plan or an attorney, for example), and a detailed log indicating to whom information was released

Standards

Information in all patient medical records is recorded in a consistent manner. Without standardization, physicians and other medical office personnel would find locating the information they need difficult and time-consuming. To ensure that medical records are well organized and easy to use, the following standards are followed at PMG:

- *Records must be clear:* Medical records should be complete and accurate. If the records are handwritten, the entries should be legible to others, made in black ink (not pencil), and dated.
- *Entries must be signed and dated:* Whether digitally entered by the provider, handwritten, or transcribed, each entry must have the signature or initials and title of the responsible provider and the date.
- *Changes must be clearly made:* An incorrect entry is marked with a single line through the words to be changed; the correct information is entered after it, so that the previous copy can be read. Corrections are also dated and signed by the person making the change. No part of a record should be otherwise altered or removed, deleted, or destroyed.

SOAP Format

The Polaris Medical Group uses *problem-oriented medical records* (POMRs) to organize patient information. The problem-oriented medical record contains a general section with data from the initial patient examination and assessment. When the patient returns for subsequent visits, the reasons for those encounters are listed separately and have their own notes. A problem-oriented medical record contains SOAP notes. In the **SOAP format** (see Figure 1-3), a patient's encounter documentation is grouped into four parts: *subjective, objective, assessment,* and *plan:*

S: The *subjective* information is based on the patient's descriptions of symptoms along with other comments.

O: The *objective* information includes the physician's descriptions of the presenting problem and data from examinations and tests.

A: The *assessment,* also called the impression or conclusion, is the physician's diagnosis, or interpretation of the subjective and objective information.

P: The *plan,* also called treatment, advice, or recommendations, includes the necessary patient monitoring, follow-up, procedures, and instructions to the patient.

This format provides an orderly system for recording clinical information about a patient encounter.

SOAP format the documentation of medical records according to *s*ubjective data, *o*bjective data, *a*ssessment, and *p*lan of treatment

---

Name: David Weatherly   Telephone: 999-555-6798

Date of Birth: 8/12/57

3/7/10   **PROBLEM 1:** Tonsillitis
         CHIEF COMPLAINT: Sore throat x2 days.

    S: Sore throat, fever, difficulty swallowing.
    O: Temperature 101°, pharyngitis with exudative tonsils.
    A: Tonsillitis.
    P: 1.   Throat culture.
         2.   1.2 units CR Bicillin.
         3.   Recheck in 10 days.

                          Robin Crebore, M.D.

3/17/10 **PROBLEM 1:** Recheck

    S: Feels better.
    O: Temperature, normal.
    A: Problem 1 resolved.
    P: Saline gargles, if necessary.

                          Robin Crebore, M.D.

FIGURE 1-3 SOAP Format

HIPAA AND PATIENT PRIVACY

Medical records are legal documents. Patients have rights to the information in their medical records. They also control the amount and type of information that is released from their records, except for the use of the data to treat them or conduct the normal business transactions of the practice.

Patient services specialists often handle requests for information from patients' medical records, and they must know what information can be released and under what circumstances. Staff members who work with a medical record are responsible for guarding the patient's privacy and confidentiality. Patient confidentiality is the basis of the physician-patient relationship. A violation of this understanding is not only a breach of trust; it may also violate federal law. The *Health Insurance Portability and Accountability Act of 1996*, known as *HIPAA*, is a federal law governing many aspects of health care, such as standards for the electronic transmission of information and the security of health care records.

HIPAA's Administrative Simplification provisions contain three rules that are important at PMG and in all medical offices:

1. The HIPAA Privacy Rule—The privacy requirements cover patients' health information.
2. The HIPAA Security Rule—The security requirements state the administrative, technical, and physical safeguards that are required to protect patients' health information.
3. The HIPAA Electronic Health Care Transactions and Code Sets—These standards require every provider who does business electronically to use the same health care transactions, code sets, and identifiers.

HIPAA Privacy Rule

The *HIPAA Privacy Rule* is the first comprehensive federal protection for the privacy of health information. These national standards protect individuals' medical records and other personal health information. The privacy rule must be followed by all health plans, health care clearinghouses, and health care providers and their business associates. The rules mandate that a provider or other group must:

- Adopt a set of privacy practices that are appropriate for its health care service's
- Notify patients about their privacy rights and how their information can be used or disclosed
- Train employees so that they understand the privacy practices

Health Insurance Portability and Accountability Act of 1996 (HIPAA) a federal law governing many aspects of health care, such as standards for the electronic transmission of information and the security of health care records

HIPAA Privacy Rule national standards that protect individuals' medical records and other personal health information

- Appoint a staff member to be the privacy official responsible for seeing that the privacy practices are adopted and followed
- Secure patient records containing individually identifiable health information so that they are not readily available to those who do not need them

Protected Health Information

The HIPAA privacy rule covers the use and disclosure of patients' **protected health information (PHI)**. PHI is defined as individually identifiable health information that is transmitted or maintained by electronic media, such as over the Internet, by computer modem, or on magnetic tape or compact disk.

Protected information includes the information below when it is used in connection with health information, such as a diagnosis or condition:

- Name
- Address (including street address, city, county, ZIP code)
- Names of relatives and employers
- Birth date
- Telephone numbers
- Fax number
- E-mail address
- Social Security number
- Medical record number
- Health plan beneficiary number
- Account number
- Certificate or license number
- Serial number of any vehicle or other device
- Website address
- Fingerprints or voiceprints
- Photographic images

Except for treatment, payment, and health care operations, the Privacy Rule limits the release of protected health information without the patient's authorization. *Treatment* means providing and coordinating the patient's medical care; *payment* refers to the exchange of information with health plans; and health care *operations* are the general business management functions. When using or disclosing protected health information at PMG, staff members must try to limit the information shared to the minimum amount necessary to accomplish the intended purpose.

protected health information (PHI) individually identifiable health information that is transmitted or maintained by electronic media, such as over the Internet, by computer modem, or on magnetic tape or compact disk

FIGURE 1-4   Page from a Notice of Privacy Practices Booklet

Notice of Privacy Practices

Under the HIPAA Privacy Rule, physician practices must provide patients with a notice of privacy practices at their first contact or encounter. This document describes the medical office's practices regarding the use and disclosure of PHI. It also establishes the office's privacy complaint procedures, explains that disclosure is limited to the minimum necessary information that is required, and discusses how consent for other types of information release is obtained. Medical practices are required to display the Notice of Privacy Practices in a prominent place in the office. To satisfy this requirement,

FIGURE 1-5 Acknowledgment of Receipt of Notice of Privacy Practices Form

Polaris Medical Group gives patients a copy of a Notice of Privacy Practices (see Figure 1-4) and asks patients to sign an Acknowledgment of Receipt of Notice of Privacy Practices, illustrated in Figure 1-5.

Authorizations

For use or disclosure other than for treatment, payment, or operations, the practice must have the patient sign an authorization to release the information. For example, information about alcohol and drug abuse may not be released without a specific authorization from the patient. The authorization document must be in plain language and include the following:

- A description of the information to be used or disclosed
- The name or other specific identification of each person authorized to use or disclose the information
- The name of the person or group of people to whom the covered entity may make the use or disclosure
- A description of each purpose of the requested use or disclosure
- An expiration date
- Signature of the individual (or authorized representative) and date

In addition, a valid authorization must include:

- A statement of the individual's right to revoke the authorization in writing
- A statement about whether the covered entity is able to base treatment, payment, enrollment, or eligibility for benefits on the authorization
- A statement that information used or disclosed after the authorization may be disclosed again by the recipient and may no longer be protected by the rule

A sample authorization form is shown in Figure 1-6.

HIPAA Security Rule

HIPAA Security Rule national standards that outline the minimum administrative, technical, and physical safeguards required to prevent unauthorized access to protected health care information

The *HIPAA Security Rule* outlines safeguards required to protect the confidentiality, integrity, and availability of health information that is stored on a computer system or that is transmitted across computer networks, including the Internet. While the HIPAA Privacy Rule applies to all forms of patients' protected health information, whether electronic, paper, or oral, the Security Rule specifically covers PHI that is created, received, maintained, or transmitted in electronic form.

The security standards are divided into three categories of safeguards: administrative, physical, and technical.

Administrative safeguards are administrative policies and procedures designed to protect electronic health information. The management of security is assigned to one individual, who conducts an assessment of the current level of data security. Once that assessment is complete, security policies and procedures are developed or modified to meet current needs. Security training is provided to educate staff members on the policies and to raise awareness of security and privacy issues.

```
                                                     MRN_____

              Authorization for Release of Patient Information

Patient Name_____      Date of Birth_____

I hereby authorize _____
              Name              Address              City        State      Zip
Telephone Number_____

to disclose the above named individual's health information as described below:

Date(s) of Service Requested (if known) or Provider: _____

Description of Information to be released: (check all that apply)
___Immunization record
___Laboratory reports                    ___Most recent history and physical
___Radiology/Imaging reports             ___Consultations
___Radiology films                       ___Progress notes
___Other_____             ___Entire medical record
                                                              _____

I understand that the information in my health record may include information relating to communicable disease, Acquired
Immunodeficiency Syndrome ("AIDS"), or Human Immunodeficiency Virus ("HIV"), behavioral or mental health,
alcohol/drug(substance) abuse or any such related information.

This information may be disclosed to and used the following individual or organization:

_____
Name              Address              City        State      Zip

Telephone Number_____

Description of the purpose of the use and/or disclosure:

___Continuing Care     ___Second Opinion       ___Social Security/Disability
___Consultation        ___Insurance
___Legal purposes      ___Personal Use
___Other: Please describe: _____

I understand that this authorization is voluntary and I may refuse to sign this authorization. I further understand that my health care
and the payment of my health care will not be affected if I do not sign this form. I understand I may inspect or copy the information to
be used or disclosed. I understand that information used or disclosed pursuant to the authorization may be subject to redisclosure by
the recipient and may no longer be protected by federal and state privacy regulations.  I understand Polaris Medical Group may
charge a processing fee for this service. I understand that this authorization will expire by law 180 days from the date of this
authorization unless I otherwise specify.  This authorization will be in effect until _____ (date or event).

I understand I may revoke this authorization at any time by notifying the Polaris Medical Group. I understand that if I revoke this
authorization I must do so in writing and the written revocation must be signed and dated with a date that is later than the date on this
authorization.  The revocation will not affect any actions taken before the receipt of the written revocation.

_____          _____
Signature of Patient or Patient's Representative    Date

_____
Printed name of Patient or Patient's Representative

_____     or   _____
Relationship to Patient                    Legal Authority (attach supporting documentation)
```

FIGURE 1-6 Sample Information Release Authorization Form

Physical safeguards are the mechanisms required to protect electronic systems, equipment, and data from threats, environmental hazards, and unauthorized intrusion. Unauthorized intrusion refers to access by individuals who do not have a need to know. For example, individuals who are not working with confidential patient information should not be able to view this type of information displayed on an office computer monitor. To prevent intrusion, PMG limits physical access to computers. A security measure can be as simple as a lock on the door or as advanced as an electronic device that requires fingerprint authentication to gain access.

Technical safeguards are the automated processes used to protect data and control access to data. Access to information is granted on an as-needed basis. For example, the individual responsible for scheduling may not need access to billing data. Examples of technical safeguards include computer passwords, antivirus and firewall software, and secure transmission systems for sending patient data from one computer to another.

Another type of technical safeguard is an ***audit trail***—an electronic log that works in the background of a computer, tracing who has accessed information and when. When new information is entered or existing data are changed, the log records the time and date of the entry as well as the name of the computer operator. The practice manager reviews the log on a regular basis to detect any irregularities or errors.

HIPAA Electronic Health Care Transactions and Code Sets

The ***HIPAA Electronic Health Care Transactions and Code Sets (TCS)*** standards are rules that make it possible for physicians and health plans to exchange electronic data using the standard format and standard codes. Under this rule, three types of standards have been set:

1. Electronic formats
2. Code sets
3. Identifiers

Electronic Formats

The HIPAA transactions standards apply to the data that are regularly sent back and forth between providers and health plans. HIPAA-covered transactions include activities such as health care claims sent by physicians and hospitals to insurance companies, payments sent by the insurance companies in response, and employee enrollment information sent by employers to their insurance companies. Each standard is labeled with both a number and a name. Either the number (such as "the 837," which is the insurance claim form) or the name (such as the "HIPAA Claim") may be used to refer to the particular electronic document format.

Code Sets

There are also standard sets of codes for diseases; treatments and procedures; and supplies or other items used to perform these actions. These standards are listed in Table 1-1.

TABLE 1-1

HIPAA Standard Code Sets for Diagnoses and Procedures

Purpose	Standard
Codes for diseases, injuries, impairments, and other health-related problems	International Classification of Diseases, Ninth Revision, Clinical Modification (ICD-9-CM), Volumes 1 and 2
Codes for procedures or other actions taken to prevent, diagnose, treat, or manage diseases, injuries, and impairments	Physicians' services: Current Procedural Terminology (CPT)
	Inpatient hospital services: International Classification of Diseases, Ninth Revision, Clinical Modification, Volume 3: Procedures
Codes for other medical services	Healthcare Common Procedure Coding System (HCPCS)

Identifiers

Identifiers are numbers of predetermined length and structure, such as a person's Social Security number. They are important for billing because the unique numbers can be used in electronic transactions. Two identifiers—for employers and for providers—have been set up by the federal government, and two—for patients and for health plans—are to be established in the future.

- The employer identifier is used to identify the patient's employer on claims. The Employer Identification Number (EIN) issued by the Internal Revenue Service is the HIPAA standard.

- The *National Provider Identifier (NPI)* is the standard unique health identifier for health care providers to use in filing health care claims and other transactions. The NPI is ten positions long, with nine numbers and a check digit. It replaces other identifying numbers that had been in use, such as the UPIN for Medicare, and eliminates the need for health care providers to use different identification numbers to identify themselves when conducting standard transactions with multiple health plans.

National Provider Identifier (NPI) a unique identifier assigned to a health care provider that is used in standard transactions, such as health care claims

Many health plans—including Medicare, Medicaid, and private health insurance issuers—and all health care clearinghouses must now accept and use NPIs in standard transactions. The numbers are assigned to individuals, such as physicians and nurses, and also to organizations, such as hospitals, pharmacies, and clinics.

Polaris Medical Group HIPAA Compliance Program

Polaris Medical Group has established a special HIPAA compliance program to help its staff members comply with HIPAA legislation. This is part of the practice's overall compliance program, which includes adherence to all government regulations, including OSHA work-safety guidelines and fair labor laws.

The practice manager, Jane Wetherall, is the compliance officer for PMG. She is responsible for:

- Training employees and new hires in all aspects of compliance
- Monitoring adherence to current policies and procedures
- Modifying policies and procedures to conform to changes in the HIPAA law

The compliance officer also establishes the procedures for employees to follow when problems are identified. Every employee is required to sign, initial, and date a compliance form at the onset of employment, to make a record for chart identification purposes in case of legal issues.

YOUR ROLE AS A PATIENT SERVICES SPECIALIST

In this text-workbook, you are the PSS at PMG. In this role, you are responsible for a variety of tasks. This section provides an overview of the types of tasks you will complete later in Part 3, On the Job.

Like most medical practices, PMG has a Policy and Procedure Manual (PPM), located in Part 2 of this text. The PPM lists the procedures that should be followed when completing the tasks in Part 3. The PPM also contains detailed information on PMG's policies. Following the guidelines in the PPM ensures that all staff members use standard methods to complete tasks.

Polaris Medical Group also maintains a set of PPMs of the insurance carriers and managed care organizations with which the practice has contracts. For your convenience, summaries of these policies and procedures can also be found in PMG's PPM.

Qualities and Attitudes of the PSS

Success as a PSS is not just about following procedures. It is also about the qualities you bring to the job and your attitude. The medical office has many things in common with other offices, but it also has unique environmental characteristics. For example, working in a medical office can be more stressful than working in other office environments because of people's reactions to illness. Some patients who come in for appointments are coping with serious illnesses or disabilities. New patients may be nervous when they see the doctor for the first time. Patients may experience a variety of emotions, ranging from fear to anger. Although the transactions you engage in (such as accepting payment from a patient) may be routine, the emotions you encounter may not be.

In the medical office, patience and enthusiasm are important qualities. It is important to appear calm in a crisis or when frustrations mount. Noise and confusion in the office create unnecessary stress for patients. To complete many of the tasks in the medical office, attention to detail is necessary. Information must be recorded with extreme accuracy. Finally, sincerity and helpfulness are always important. Be willing to assist other staff members not only when asked, but also whenever the opportunity arises.

General Responsibilities

Polaris Medical Group has identified the general responsibilities that are expected of every employee regardless of position.

All staff members must:

- Arrive at the office on time and stay until the end of the shift
- Return from breaks and meals on time
- Follow office procedures and report issues concerning safety, infection control, and exposure control
- Observe and follow all office policies, especially those related to confidentiality
- Dress in a neat and appropriate style, with their identification tags visible at all times
- Demonstrate effective verbal and written communication skills
- Demonstrate their willingness to work cooperatively with all patients and coworkers
- Interact with patients without prejudice with regard to age, gender, race, creed, and disability
- Organize and prioritize their workloads in an efficient manner
- Follow verbal and written instructions from supervisors, managers, and physicians
- Maintain neat and legible records and documentation
- Seek the advice of a supervisor when the proper or correct course of action is not clear

- Adapt quickly to changes in the work environment or schedule
- Learn new concepts and procedures as necessary
- Juggle more than one task at a time when necessary
- Complete work assignments within a reasonable time frame

Your Typical Day at Polaris Medical Group

Each day, you will perform a variety of tasks. For example, you will interact with patients on the telephone and in the office. You will work on the office computer network to complete scheduling and billing tasks. You will look up information in medical records or in the PPM when necessary. The following sections describe the specific responsibilities of your position.

Scheduling Patients for Appointments   Patients call the office to schedule new appointments or reschedule existing appointments. Scheduling tasks include:

- Scheduling, rescheduling, and canceling appointments
- Adding patients to the recall list as appropriate
- Maintaining computerized office schedules for physicians, including patient appointments, professional obligations, and personal time off
- Printing copies of the day's schedule as soon as you arrive in the office in the morning; distributing copies to physicians and staff members; and maintaining an up-to-date schedule on the computer
- On a weekly basis, generating a patient recall list
- On a daily basis, calling patients on the recall list to schedule appointments

Recording and Maintaining Patient Information   When a patient comes to PMG for the first time, information is collected and recorded in the medical record and in the computer. Similarly, patient records are updated each time the patient phones or visits the office. The patient information tasks include:

- Gathering and recording information from a new patient over the telephone at the time the appointment is made
- Asking new patients to fill out the patient information form (PIF) when they arrive in the office, and reviewing it for completeness, paying particular attention to the insurance section
- Distributing the Notice of Privacy Practices form to each patient, and asking the patient to sign, date, and return the Acknowledgment of Receipt of Privacy Practices form
- Asking to see the patient's insurance identification card, photocopying the front and back of the card, and filing the copy in the patient's medical record

- Inputting data from the PIF and the insurance card (if appropriate) into the computer
- Asking a patient whose information (such as employer, insurance, or address) has changed since his or her last visit to complete a new PIF, and recording changes in the computer the same day, before new charges are entered
- Recording information gathered during patient phone calls regarding changes in address, employment, insurance carrier, marital status, and so on
- Reading and storing e-mail messages

Maintaining Third-Party Payer Information Information is recorded and updated regarding each patient's insurance carrier or managed care organization. Information about each specific health plan is also recorded. Summary information about the major insurance plans in which PMG participates is listed in the PPM. To produce accurate claims, you must be familiar with the requirements of each third-party payer. Tasks include:

- Looking up payer information for each patient as needed
- Verifying each patient's insurance eligibility
- Collecting a copayment from the patient at the time of the visit if the patient's insurance plan has a copayment requirement
- Checking with patients who are participants in managed care plans to see if they need referrals before they can be seen by one of the physicians at PMG; if a referral is needed, checking for a proper referral or contacting the office of the patient's primary care physician for the necessary information
- Checking for proper preauthorization; if preauthorization is required, contacting the health plan to obtain a preauthorization number
- Recording referral information in the computer
- Recording preauthorization numbers in the computer

Educating Patients and Responding to Patient Inquiries Educating patients often includes informing them about charges and the payment process in general. Some patients do not understand the fees. If the planned services are expected to be costly and are not covered by the patient's insurance, it is PMG's policy to discuss these charges with the patient before the services are provided. In addition, patients sometimes call or stop by the office to inquire about the status of a particular insurance claim or to ask about an account balance. You are responsible for researching the account and responding to the patient's question in a timely manner. This involves:

- Researching and resolving patient inquiries regarding services, billing, or charges
- Using relevant information to determine the validity of the inquiry and the source of the error, if there is one
- Contacting the patient to communicate the resolution of the problem

Recording Charges, Payments, and Adjustments at the Time of an Encounter Every time a PMG physician sees a patient at the office, hospital, or nursing home, a service is performed, and a charge needs to be recorded. Similarly, any payments received from patients must be recorded. Adjustments are required when there is a difference between the amount charged and the amount that is accepted as payment.

A new billing tool for collectiing payment at the time of service is known as *real-time claims adjudication (RTCA)*. Increasingly used in computerized offices, RTCA is likely the billing model that will be the most widely implemented in the future. With RTCA, a billing assistant submits claims at the time the patient checks out. Once a claim is submitted, assuming the payer has RTCA capabilities, the payor's computer system adjudicates the claim within minutes and sends back an EOB. The billing assistant then discusses the payer's decision with the patient in person, and the patient pays any balance due before leaving. If there is a problem with the claim, such as missing information, the billing assistant can work with the patient to resolve the problem and resubmit the claim. The only follow up for the medical office is to verify that the payer's portion of the payment is received. Payment usually follows within twenty-four hours.

Regardless of whether a medical office uses RTCA or some other form of collecting payments at the time of an encounter, the billing tasks include:

- Preparing encounter forms at the beginning of each day for all patients with appointments
- At the conclusion of an office visit:
  - Reviewing charges with the patient
  - Recording charges on the encounter form and then entering them in the computer
  - Estimating the patient's financial responsibility
  - Collecting payments as appropriate; for example, deductibles, payments for noncovered services, or balances due. (*Note:* Depending on the particular health plan, some patients do not make payments at the time of office visits, but are instead billed for the balance after the remittance advice [RA] from the plan has arrived.)

- Recording the amount of payment and type of payment (such as check or credit card) on the encounter form, entering the information in the computer, and applying the payment to the proper charge(s)
- Thanking patients for their payments, and generating walkout receipts at the time payment is received or upon request

Generating Health Care Claims   Timely submission of claims helps solidify the finances of the practice. The sooner claims are created and submitted, the sooner payment arrives. It is your responsibility to prepare health care claims. If a claim is rejected, you must discover whether an error was made and, if so, resubmit the claim as soon as possible. Claim tasks include:

- Generating health care claims and checking all claims for accuracy before submission, including:
  - Diagnosis and procedure code compliance
  - Correct linkage of diagnoses and procedures
  - Medical necessity of procedures
  - Billing compliance—making sure the charges are billable according to the payer's conditions
- Reviewing claim acknowledgments to verify that claims have been received
- Preparing claim status reports on a weekly basis

Monitoring Payments from Third-Party Payers   Once a third-party payer makes a decision on a claim, you are responsible for checking the results. This includes:

- Comparing the information on the RA with the expected payment
- If a claim is denied, reduced, or overpaid, researching the reason and resolving any discrepancies regarding services or billing, analyzing relevant information to determine the validity of the payer's decision or the source of an error, if there is one, and contacting the payer to resolve the problem
- Appealing denied or rejected claims as necessary
- Posting payments to patients' accounts
- Contacting the payer if a claim is not paid within thirty days; following up on and/or resubmitting the claim as necessary

Generating Patient Statements and Financial Reports   It is important to prepare and print patient statements regularly for billing. In addition, the financial transactions of the medical practice must also be reported daily, weekly, and monthly. Patient day sheets summarize the number of patients seen by the physicians on a given day, the procedures performed, the charges and payments for the day, and other information. Reports that are generated on a weekly or monthly basis include patient and insurance aging reports.

Collecting Overdue Payments from Patients An unpaid account with a balance that is thirty days past due is considered overdue. It is usually the job of the PSS to collect payments on patients' overdue accounts. Each week, the PSS generates an aging report showing which patients' accounts are overdue ("aged") and by how many days. The report indicates whether the account is thirty, sixty, or ninety days past due. Generally if the account is thirty days past due, the PSS sends out a reminder notice or a second statement or phones the patient about the payment.

In some cases, or for large amounts, the office may decide to extend credit to a patient by setting up a payment plan. Usually the agreement is to divide the bill over a period of months, with the patient making regular monthly payments. Finance charges may or may not be applied. In the case of Polaris Medical Group, finance charges are not applied to the payment plan.

At Polaris Medical Group, when an account is ninety days overdue, the PSS generates a collection letter. If a patient does not respond, additional collection letters are sent. Ultimately if the office's collection procedures fail, an office may hire an outside collection agency to pursue the matter, or the office may decide that the account is uncollectible and write off the uncollected amount as a bad debt. Future services for patients with such accounts are usually on a cash-only basis. It is the job of the PSS to keep track of where an account is in the collection process and to follow up on collections on a weekly basis.

Updating CPT and ICD-9-CM Codes in the Database The *Current Procedural Terminology* (CPT) and *International Classification of Diseases* (ICD-9-CM) codes are updated annually. New codes are added; existing codes are modified; and old codes are marked inactive. When the practice manager requests it, these changes must be made by the PSS to PMG's computer database.

For questions 1 through 6, write the letter that corresponds to the correct answer in the space provided.

_____ 1. An internist specializes in treating:
    a. patients of all ages
    b. adults
    c. diseases of the organs
    d. families

_____ 2. Physicians responsible for overseeing patients' overall health care and for referring patients to specialists are known as:
    a. family practitioners
    b. primary care physicians
    c. internists
    d. family care physicians

_____ 3. Which of the following is generally not part of a patient's medical record?
    a. insurance correspondence
    b. chart notes
    c. patient information form
    d. remittance advice (RA)

_____ 4. The HIPAA security standards are divided into which three categories:
    a. electronic, paper, and oral
    b. Internet, PHI, and networks
    c. confidentiality, integrity, and availability
    d. administrative, physical, and technical

_____ 5. The *O* in SOAP refers to:
    a. obstetrical
    b. observation
    c. objective
    d. ordinary

_____ 6. The HIPAA compliance program is a set of policies and procedures that helps medical office employees:
    a. comply with laws and regulations and avoid misconduct
    b. adhere to personnel conduct standards set by the practice
    c. achieve the lowest percentage of rejected insurance claims
    d. respond to patient billing inquiries in a standardized manner

Indicate whether items 7 through 15 are true or false by writing "T" or "F" in the blank provided.

_____ 7. Medical records cannot be released under any circumstances without the written consent of the patient.

_____ 8. Any medical office employee who works with a patient's medical record is responsible for safeguarding the patient's privacy and confidentiality.

_____ 9. Passwords and firewalls are examples of administrative safeguards used to protect electronic health information.

_____ 10. The NPI is a unique identifier that is used to identify the patient's employer on health care claims and other HIPAA transactions.

_____ 11. One of the responsibilities of the patient services specialist (PSS) is maintaining computerized schedules for Polaris Medical Group physicians.

_____ 12. A new patient should be asked to complete a patient information form during the first visit to the office.

_____ 13. The PSS is not responsible for educating patients about Polaris Medical Group's fees and payment procedures.

_____ 14. At the conclusion of a patient's office visit, the PSS collects the payment or copayment from the patient and records this information on the encounter form.

_____ 15. At Polaris Medical Group, the PSS begins sending out collection letters when payments are thirty days past due.

Part 2

Polaris Medical Group Policy and Procedure Manual

The Policy and Procedure Manual (PPM) provides staff members with information about the practice's general policies. It also covers the specific procedures that you are expected to follow while employed as a patient services specialist at Polaris Medical Group. The PPM contains detailed guidelines on the way the practice processes new patient registration, referrals, appointment scheduling, billing, and payments.

Read the PPM before proceeding with your work in Part 3. After you have read the PPM, sign in the box at the bottom of page 26. Then, as you work through the daily assignments in Part 3, refer to the PPM as needed.

LEARNING OUTCOMES

After successfully completing Part 2, you will be able to define the key terms and:

2.1 Locate the practice's contact information.

2.2 Discuss employee rights that are ensured.

2.3 Describe employment policies.

2.4 Discuss routine and emergency telephone procedures.

2.5 Identify the procedures for appointment scheduling and office visits.

2.6 Discuss the practice's patient privacy guidelines.

2.7 Describe the policies and procedures for payment for services, billing, reviewing remittance advices, and handling collections and patient billing disputes.

2.8 List the required daily logs.

2.9 Compare the guidelines for Medicare, Medicaid, and workers' compensation health care claims.

KEY TERMS

COBRA

grievance

medical necessity

Medigap insurance

preauthorization

Universal Precautions

workers' compensation insurance

Reading Acknowledgment

The PPM is not an employment contract. Polaris Medical Group makes every attempt to offer secure employment and rewarding careers to its employees. However, PMG makes no guarantee of length of employment or possible advancement. Length of employment and pace of advancement are related to a number of factors, including your adherence to the standards of performance and conduct contained in this PPM. Thus, all employees of PMG are employed for an unspecified length of time, and employment may be terminated at any time at the will of either the employee or the practice.

Polaris Medical Group reserves the right to alter or deviate from these policies and procedures from time to time as is necessary.

I have read and understood Polaris Medical Group's Policy and Procedure Manual. (Sign after reading entire PPM.)

_____   _____
                Employee's Signature   Date

CONTENTS

PRACTICE INFORMATION

The first section of the PPM provides information about the practice, the physicians and staff, the referring physician, the hospital and nursing home with which the practice is affiliated, and the laboratory service it uses.

Polaris Medical Group
Address: 2100 Grace Avenue, Columbus, OH 43214
Phone: 999-555-9800
Fax: 999-555-9801
Office Hours: 9:00 A.M. to 5:00 P.M., Monday through Friday

Personnel
Physician: Robin C. Crebore, M.D., F.A.A.F.P., NPI 1145678922
Beeper Number: 999-666-9436

Physician: Michael P. Mahabir, M.D., F.A.C.P., NPI 2167891336
Beeper Number: 999-666-9756

Practice Manager: Jane Wetherall
Physician's Assistant: Michelle Maligo
Medical Laboratory Technician: Thomas Bouck
Bookkeeper: Joseph Lambert
Patient Services Specialist: _____ (your name)

Accounting Firm
Name: Marilyn M. Chan, Chan and Grimwald
Address: 9000 South Street, Cincinnati, OH 43214
Phone: 999-555-6060
Fax: 999-555-6061

Referring Physician
Name: Rachel P. Innanni, M.D., F.A.A.F.P., NPI 5211361139
Facility: Rennsit Clinic
Address: 98 Broadway, Columbus, OH 43214
Phone: 800-555-1920
Fax: 800-555-1212
Medicare Participating: Yes

Hospital Affiliation
Name: St. Mary's
Address: 2500 Grace Avenue, Columbus OH 43214
Phone: 999-555-0001
Fax: 999-555-0002

Nursing Home Affiliation
Name: Grandview Home
Address: 300 Center Street, Grandview, OH 46757
Phone: 999-555-1010
Fax: 999-555-1011
Contact Person: Louise Schroth
Extension: 325

Laboratory Services
Name: Medco
Address: 1415 Central Avenue, Columbus, OH 43214
Phone: 999-555-8989
Fax: 999-555-8990
Contact Person: John Witkowski
Extension: 1014
Medicare Participating: Yes

Emergency Phone Numbers
Local Emergency Police/Fire/Ambulance: 911
Local Poison Control Center: 999-777-0000

EQUAL EMPLOYMENT OPPORTUNITY, NONDISCRIMINATION, AND AFFIRMATIVE ACTION STATEMENT

Polaris Medical Group does not discriminate on the basis of race, color, age, sex, national origin, religion, creed, or disability in the admission or access to, or treatment or employment of, its programs and activities. The practice manager has been designated as the Human Resource Coordinator to coordinate all efforts to comply with section 504 of the Rehabilitation Act of 1973 and its implementing regulation that prohibits discrimination on the basis of disability.

The clinic is an equal opportunity employer. All applicants for employment will be considered. All persons employed, including management staff, professionals, technicians, and others, will be treated without regard to age, race, color, religion, sex, national origin, handicap, or disability. Such action includes, but is not limited to, the following:

- Employment, promotion, demotion, transfers, layoffs, and termination
- Recruitment and recruitment advertising

- Rates of pay and other forms of compensation
- Training opportunities
- Practice-sponsored social and recreational programs

All employees are responsible for reporting perceived illegal discrimination to the practice manager.

TYPES OF EMPLOYMENT

PMG classifies employees in the following categories:

- *Regular full-time employee:* An employee who is regularly scheduled for at least forty hours a week and who has worked for more than three months. Eligible for benefits.

- *Trial work period full-time employee:* An employee who is regularly scheduled for a least forty hours a week and who has not yet worked for three months. Does not receive benefits.

- *Temporary full-time employee:* An employee who is regularly scheduled for at least forty hours a week and whose length of employment will be less than six months. Does not receive benefits.

- *Regular part-time employee:* An employee who is regularly scheduled for less than forty hours a week and who has worked for more than three months. Does not receive benefits.

- *Trial work period part-time employee:* An employee who is regularly scheduled for less than forty hours a week and who has not yet worked for three months. Does not receive benefits.

- *Temporary part-time employee:* An employee who is regularly scheduled to work less than forty hours a week and whose length of employment will be less than six months. Does not receive benefits.

WAGES AND COMPENSATION

Polaris Medical Group's policy is that wage compensation will be in accordance with the Fair Labor Standards Act (FLSA) and state law. Some employees and occupations are considered exempt from additional payment for working more than forty hours in a week. The practice manager determines which employees are exempt and which are nonexempt.

Pay Rates

Polaris Medical Group compensates all employees with at least the federal minimum wage, or the state minimum wage if it is higher, for each hour of work performed voluntarily. Rates are based on:

- Job performance
- Length of employment
- Additional qualifications, education, or certifications
- Prior salary history

Overtime Compensation

All overtime must be approved by management before it is worked. If overtime is not preapproved, the employee may be disallowed those hours and not compensated. Employees who are considered nonexempt are entitled to overtime pay at the rate of not less than one-and-a half times their regular pay for any portion of hours worked in excess of forty hours in a single workweek.

If the forty-hour requirement has not yet been met, an employee will not be paid overtime for hours in excess of eight per day or for work on Saturdays, Sundays, holidays, or regular days of rest. Any overtime compensation earned during a specific pay cycle will be paid on the regular payday for the period in which that pay cycle ends.

Pay Dates

Pay dates for the current year are posted on the bulletin board. Checks will be available at 9:00 A.M. on the dates listed. Employees who need to obtain their checks early must contact the practice manager at least three working days in advance.

Employee Time Records

Nonexempt employees will be responsible for clocking in and out on a time card. The time card serves as a permanent record of the time worked. An error on the time card must be immediately reported and corrected in the same week in which the error occurred. At the end of the pay period, time cards are submitted to the practice manager. Falsification of a time card will be grounds for immediate dismissal.

Employees record their own starting and ending times on their own time cards. Clocking in or out for another employee will be grounds for progressive disciplinary action, beginning with verbal reprimand, to written reprimand, to suspension, and finally to termination.

All nonexempt employees are required to clock out for a one-hour lunch during shifts of five hours or more. Employees are not allowed to skip this lunch break without approval. Failure to clock out for lunch break will result in progressive disciplinary action.

An employee who needs to leave the clinic on personal business is required to clock out before leaving. Failure to do so will result in progressive disciplinary action.

Repeated failure to clock in or out at the beginning or end of a shift, when leaving for or returning from lunch, or when leaving for or returning from personal business will result in progressive disciplinary action.

Performance Evaluations

Performance evaluations are conducted at three months, twelve months, and each year thereafter, or more often if necessary. Reviews are held annually on the employee's anniversary date. The practice manager will prepare the evaluation and discuss it with the employee. The employee will be given an opportunity to ask questions and discuss matters of concern. The practice manager and the employee will sign the evaluation at the completion of the review. All evaluations become part of the employee's permanent personnel file.

A review of salary and wages may also occur during the performance evaluation. Pay increases are not automatic. If an increase is recommended, it will be in accordance with approved scheduled wages, unless otherwise authorized. Increases become effective the first pay period after the anniversary date.

Employee Benefits

Below are some of the benefits offered by PMG to regular full-time employees. Employees are advised to consult with the practice manager for a comprehensive description of available benefits.

- Employee assistance program
- Health service program
- Medical/health insurance
- Professional liability insurance
- Workers' compensation insurance
- Unemployment insurance
- Paid holidays
- Credit union membership
- Investment, retirement, or pension plans

- Severance pay
- Short-term/long-term disability
- Personal time off/personal emergency leave
- Tuition reimbursement
- Paid continuing education/reimbursement for continuing education
- Paid time off for jury duty
- Military leave/time off for active reserve or National Guard duty
- Paid time off for death in immediate family/bereavement
- Maternity leave
- Paid vacation time
- Paid sick time
- Family leave
- Compensatory time off

Employee Grievances

grievance a job-related problem that an employee feels should be corrected

A *grievance* related to discrimination based on race, color, sex, age, creed, marital status, national origin, or disability is processed in accordance with the nondiscrimination grievance procedure described below.

A grievance procedure must be initiated within ten days of the incident. No employee is criticized or penalized in any way for using the grievance procedure; it is the means of resolving an employee problem when normal conversation between an employee and supervisor cannot resolve the problem. Employees and supervisors alike should consider this procedure as another part of PMG's management of open communication. All employee grievance discussions are strictly confidential.

In order to provide the employee with a means of expressing dissatisfaction relating to wages, hours of work, administration of personnel policies and procedures, and perceived unfair or inequitable treatment or discipline or other conditions of employment, PMG has adopted the following grievance procedure:

1. The employee should talk over the problem with the practice manager within ten working days of the date of the problem.

2. If the problem is not resolved informally, the employee must submit a written statement describing the situation, with dates and signatures, to the practice manager.

3. Within five working days, the practice manager, the employee, and one of the physicians will meet to discuss, and attempt to resolve, the situation. The physician's decision will be final and binding.

RESIGNATION, TERMINATION, DISCHARGE, AND COBRA BENEFITS

Polaris Medical Group has specific written policies regarding resignation, termination, discharge, and COBRA benefits. This section of the manual provides an overview of these policies. For a complete copy of the policies, ask the practice manager.

Resignation

When an employee decides to end employment with PMG, advance notice of one month is requested from all managers, supervisors, and registered/licensed personnel. All other employees are requested to give two weeks' notice. Once a resignation notice from an employee is received, management reserves the right to allow the employee to continue employment to the resignation date or to accept the date of notice as the employee's last date of employment. All resignations are to be submitted in writing to the practice manager.

Termination

In some instances, termination may be initiated by management for nondisciplinary reasons including, but not limited, to the following:

- Work assignment completed (temporary employee)
- Workforce reduction
- Position abolished; employee cannot be transferred to another position
- Workload decreased or work assignments changed

Discharge

Discharge is immediate dismissal for misconduct. No advance notice is given, and terminal pay covers only the time actually worked prior to discharge.

COBRA Benefits

The Consolidated Omnibus Reconciliation Act of 1986 *(COBRA)*, also known as Public Law 99-272, states that an employer is required to provide continuation of group plan health insurance to terminated employees and other qualified beneficiaries for a period of up to eighteen months. Any employee eligible for PMG benefits is also eligible for COBRA benefits. Beneficiaries are generally required to pay the entire premium for the coverage.

COBRA   federal legislation requiring an employer with twenty or more employees that sponsors a group health benefit plan to continue health insurance coverage of terminated employees and other qualified beneficiaries for a period of up to eighteen months

PERSONNEL CONDUCT ISSUES

Polaris Medical Group has developed guidelines for employee conduct while on the job. The following section of the PPM provides an overview of these guidelines.

Contributions and Solicitations

Solicitations or distribution of printed material by employees and/or visitors for purposes other than an officially approved program are prohibited. Such unapproved action by an employee will be considered grounds for progressive disciplinary action.

Identification Badges

In order to readily identify all staff members to our patients and visitors, identification (ID) badges must be worn at all times during working hours. This creates an atmosphere of professionalism, courtesy, and efficiency. The employee ID badge is clinic property and must be turned in to the practice manager upon resignation or termination. The final paycheck will not be given to the employee until the badge is received.

Inclement Weather

Polaris Medical Group does not close during adverse weather conditions. Each employee should determine whether it is safe to travel to work. Employees are expected to make an attempt to report to work. Notify the practice if you are unable to arrive at work at the normal time. Those who are unable to report to work will not be paid unless they substitute vacation or other paid time off for the time missed.

Sexual Harassment

Sexual harassment is a form of discrimination prohibited by Title VII of the Civil Rights Act of 1964. It is defined by the Equal Employment Opportunity Commission as: "unwelcome sexual advances, requests for sexual favors, and other verbal or physical conduct of a sexual nature when submission to the conduct enters into employment decisions and/or the conduct unreasonably interferes with an individual's work performance or creates an intimidating, hostile, or offensive working environment."

Polaris Medical Group does not tolerate verbal or physical conduct by any employee that harasses, disrupts, or interferes with another employee's work performance or that creates an intimidating, offensive, or hostile environment. Prohibited behavior includes:

- Sexual flirtations, touching, advances, or propositions
- Verbal abuse of a sexual nature
- Graphic or suggestive comments about an individual's dress or body
- The use of sexually degrading words to describe an individual
- The display in the workplace of sexually suggestive objects or pictures

Any employee who believes that the actions or words of a supervisor or employee constitute sexual harassment must immediately report the incident to the practice manager. The complaint will be taken seriously and investigated immediately. If an employee is not satisfied with the handling of a complaint or the action taken, the employee should bring the complaint to the attention of a physician. In all cases, the employee will be informed of the ongoing findings and conclusion.

Any employee, supervisor, or manager who is found to have engaged in the harassment of another individual, whether coworker, patient, vendor, or anyone else, will be subject to progressive disciplinary action, up to and including termination.

Dress Code

Employees are expected to appear neat, clean, and well groomed at all times. It is important for employees to be aware that patients and visitors may judge the entire practice and the attention they receive on the basis of the personal appearance of an employee. Employees are expected to use good judgment and moderation in dress and grooming at all times while on the job. Employees whose appearance is not acceptable in a conservative, professional environment, or whose attire represents a safety hazard, are subject to progressive disciplinary action.

Smoking and Tobacco Use

In order to promote the health and well-being of patients, visitors, and employees, no cigarettes or tobacco products of any kind are allowed inside the building or in the parking lot. Personnel found smoking or using tobacco will be subject to progressive disciplinary action.

Substance Abuse

It is the duty of PMG to provide a safe work environment in accordance with the Drug-Free Workplace Act of 1988. While the intention is not to intrude on the private lives of employees, the concern that chemical-substance use that might affect job competence, public or employee safety, public trust, or the practice's reputation requires adherence to the following policy.

Illegal use or working under the influence of alcohol, illegal drugs, or prescription drugs (to the extent that work performance is affected) will not be tolerated. The purpose of any drug testing conducted is to ensure that public safety and the personal safety of employees and patients are not endangered as a result of drug use by employees and that all employees perform their jobs both efficiently and in a manner to promote public trust. Violations of this policy will result in disciplinary action up to and including termination and may also have legal consequences.

Personal Telephone Calls and Visits

Personal telephone calls and visits to employees must be kept to a minimum and must not interfere with an employee's work. It is not appropriate for employees to receive personal visits while working. Personal visits should take place after work hours and away from the clinic.

Phone calls to arrange transportation and check on the safety of immediate family members, as well as other important outgoing calls, may be made. These calls should be local calls and should be made during breaks or lunch periods. Incoming calls should be kept to a minimum and restricted primarily to emergency messages. Employees whose work is frequently interrupted by personal calls or visits may be subject to progressive disciplinary action.

Personal Use of Computers and E-mail

The Polaris Medical Group e-mail system belongs to the medical group. Staff members are permitted access to the computer system to assist them in the performance of their jobs. Personal use of the computer system is prohibited if the use interferes with the user's or any other employee's work performance; has a negative effect on the operation of the computer system; or violates any other provision of this policy or any other policy of the Polaris Medical Group.

The e-mail system may not be used for unlawful activities or for commercial purposes that are not directly related to the practice's business. Prohibited uses of e-mail include but are not limited to:

- Sending commercial advertisements, solicitations, or promotions
- Sending destructive programs such as computer viruses
- Sending copies of documents in violation of copyright laws

- Using e-mail to harass, intimidate, defame, or discriminate against others or to interfere with the ability of others to conduct business

- Using e-mail for any purpose restricted or prohibited by laws or PMG policies

- Constructing an e-mail communication so it appears to be from someone else

- Accessing electronic mail without authorization, breaching security measures on any electronic mail system, or intercepting electronic mail transmissions without authorization

Universal Precautions

All employees are required to utilize the Centers for Disease Control and Prevention (CDC)-approved Universal Precaution techniques while performing patient care functions. *Universal Precautions* are specific techniques designed to prevent health care workers from exposing themselves and others to infection by pathogens, such as the human immunodeficiency virus (HIV).

Universal Precautions techniques issued by the Centers for Disease Control and Prevention (CDC) to protect health care workers from infection

OFFICE HOURS AND ATTENDANCE

The normal hours of operation are 9:00 A.M. to 5:00 P.M., Monday through Friday. Working additional hours outside the normal range will sometimes be necessary. This is not a common occurrence, but when it does become necessary, all employees are expected to be available to work.

During each workday, you are allowed two fifteen-minute breaks. These breaks are usually taken at regularly scheduled times. The practice manager will determine the schedule of breaks. A staff member who works a five-hour day or longer is required to take a one-hour lunch break.

Staff members who work on a part-time basis must clock in at the beginning of each shift and clock out at the end of each shift. In addition, they should not clock in more than fifteen minutes prior to their regular start time. When a part-time staff member works more than five hours, he or she should clock out for a one-hour lunch break. Part-time personnel should not exceed eight hours per day or forty hours per week. These regulations should be followed without deviation unless authorization is given by the practice manager. All overtime requires prior approval from the practice manager.

Employees are hired to perform certain duties in the medical office during a specified time period. For patients to receive quality care and for the practice to run efficiently, all staff members must be present. One employee's lateness or absence can disrupt the efficient functioning of the entire practice. For this reason, PMG has developed an attendance policy. While we recognize that everyone has an occasional emergency that prevents on-time arrival at the office (for example, an automobile breakdown or a family illness), we expect all employees to be at work when they are scheduled.

Definitions of Absences

Scheduled Absences   Holidays, vacation days, and other days off, scheduled in advance and approved by the practice manager, are considered scheduled absences.

Unscheduled Absences   Failure to be present during scheduled working hours, during overtime hours, or at a required class or meeting is considered an unscheduled absence.

Lateness/Leaving Early   Employees are considered late if they arrive more than ten minutes after the scheduled start of their shift. Employees are considered to have left early if they leave the office before the scheduled end of their shift.

Excused Absences   The following are considered excused absences:

- Scheduled absences
- Absences that have been preapproved by the practice manager
- Absences or lateness on a day the practice has defined as a weather-related emergency
- Absences for assigned jury duty
- Absences due to the death of a family member
- Other absences as defined by the practice manager

Unexcused Absences   The following are considered unexcused absences:

- Unscheduled absences or lateness
- Absences without proper notification (for example, having a friend or family member call in to report your absence)
- Late arrivals or early departures to and from work
- Other absences as defined by the practice manager

Attendance Policy

The key elements of PMG's attendance policy are:

- All employees are expected to be at the office during their assigned work hours.

- An employee who is not at work during the required period must have prior authorization from the practice manager.

- Employees are not permitted to leave the building except during their lunch breaks without prior approval from the practice manager.

- All employees should inform the practice manager as far in advance as possible of any known reasons for lateness or absence. It is not appropriate to have a family member or friend call in and speak to the practice manager. This discussion must take place between the employee and the practice manager.

- If advance notice is given and the practice manager does not approve the lateness or absence, and if the time is taken anyway, it will be considered an unexcused absence.

- The first incidence of an unexcused absence results in a written notation in the employee's personnel file. The second incident of an unexcused absence results in immediate dismissal.

- Any absences that occur during an employee's ninety-day probationary period will not be paid except in the case of illness.

- An employee who is not at work for two consecutive days without informing the practice manager will be subject to immediate dismissal.

- An employee who is absent two or more consecutive days due to illness will be required to present a medical note from a physician upon returning to work. If such a document is not submitted, the employee will not be paid for the time.

TELEPHONE PROCEDURES

The voice on the other end of the telephone is often the first contact patients have with the practice. Callers form impressions about the office as a whole based on the nature of the phone call and the tone of voice of the person answering the phone. For this reason, it is very important to sound calm, friendly, and efficient when answering the phone. Even if you are having a stressful day, it is important to not sound that way on the telephone.

The patient services specialist is responsible for answering the telephone. As in all medical offices, the telephone should be answered promptly. There is always the possibility that a call is an emergency. The proper way to answer the phone is "Polaris Medical Group, this is _____ (your name). May I help you?"

Documenting Telephone Calls

Physicians must keep records of all telephone conversations with patients. These notes are stored in the patients' medical records. The patient services specialist must also document telephone calls with patients that involve requests for appointments or complaints.

Screening Telephone Calls

The practice receives a variety of telephone calls throughout the day. Common types of calls relate to:

- Appointments
- Billing questions
- Insurance questions
- General office questions, such as office hours
- Requests for prescription renewals
- Reports from outside labs or X-ray sites
- Reports from a hospital concerning a patient's condition
- Reports from a patient concerning his or her condition
- Referral requests

All calls must be screened before they are transferred within the office. To determine whether the call should be transferred and who should receive it, certain information should first be obtained from the caller:

1. Determine who the caller is (patient, family member of patient, physician, pharmacist, insurance claim specialist, and so on).
2. Determine what the call is about (billing question, lab report, referral, and so on). (See below and pages 43–45 for information concerning what to do in the case of an emergency call.)
3. Decide whether to transfer the call. Using the information obtained in steps 1 and 2, review Table 2-1 and make a decision about whether to put the call through to the appropriate person.
4. Put emergency calls through to a physician immediately. If neither physician is available, seek the advice of your manager. You may need to suggest that the patient go to the emergency room or to another physician's office.

Taking Telephone Messages

Sometimes you will need to take a message rather than transfer the call. This usually happens when the call is for a staff member who is unable to take the

TABLE 2-1

Polaris Medical Group
Telephone Routing Chart

Type of Call	Transfer to Physician	Take Message for Physician	Route to Personnel Listed
Emergency	X		
Other physician	if possible		
Appointments			PSS
Patient billing or insurance inquiry			PSS
Patient progress report		X	
Patient request for test results		X	
Prescription renewals		X	
Patient questions about medication		X	
Office business			Practice manager
Personal calls for physicians		X	
Business calls			Practice manager
Personal call for others			Appropriate personnel

call at that time. When taking a telephone message, write down the following information:

- Name of person calling
- Patient's name
- Date and time of the call
- The caller's phone number
- Reason for the call
- Name of person who took the call
- How urgent the call is—that is, whether the call needs to be returned, is for someone's information only, and so on

Handling Emergency Telephone Calls

During the course of the day, patients may call the office with emergencies. The following procedures must be followed when an emergency call is taken:

1. Remain calm. You will be better able to assist the patient if you remain calm and focused on the problem.

2. Obtain the following information:
   - Name of the caller
   - Caller's relationship to the patient (if the caller is not the patient)
   - Patient's name
   - Patient's age
   - Patient's detailed symptoms or complaints and the duration of those symptoms
   - If the call is about an accident or injury, a description of how the accident or injury occurred
   - Patient's reaction to the situation
   - Description of any treatment that has been given
   - Caller's name and the phone number and address where the patient is located

3. Summarize the information and speak it back to the caller to confirm that you have heard and understood the situation.

4. Refer to PMG's list of symptoms and complaints that require emergency attention to determine whether this situation requires immediate action.

5. If the situation is a medical emergency, immediately transfer the call to a physician. If neither of the physicians is available, put the caller on hold, and discuss the situation with the practice manager.

6. If the situation is not a medical emergency, schedule the patient for an appointment as soon as possible.

Symptoms/Complaints Considered Emergencies   The following symptoms and complaints are handled as emergency calls:

- Loss of consciousness
- Lack of breathing or difficulty breathing
- Symptoms of a heart attack, including severe chest pain or pressure; pain radiating from the chest to the arm, neck, shoulder, jaw, back, or abdomen; nausea or vomiting; shortness of breath; weakness; pale skin color
- Symptoms of a stroke, including severe headache, slurred speech, dizziness
- Symptoms of shock, including feeling faint; sweating; pale skin color; weakness; rapid pulse; cold, moist skin; drowsiness or confusion
- Severe bleeding
- Pain or pressure in the abdomen that does not cease
- Severe vomiting

- Bloody stools

- Severe swelling/edema of extremities

- Poisoning

- Electrical shock

- Drowning

- Snake bites

- Injuries from an automobile accident

- Back, head, or neck injuries

- Broken bones

- Allergic reactions to foods or insect bites or stings

- Chemicals or foreign objects in the eye

- Severe burns or injuries from an explosion

- Deep bites from humans or animals

- Symptoms of sunstroke, including loss of consciousness or confusion; strong, rapid pulse; flushed skin that is hot and dry

- Symptoms of hypothermia, including slurred speech; becoming increasingly clumsy, irritable, confused, unreasonable, and tired; being in a coma with slow, weak breathing and heartbeat

PATIENT PRIVACY AND CONFIDENTIALITY PROCEDURES

You are required to maintain a patient's privacy and to safeguard the protected health information (PHI) of anyone who receives services at PMG. Patient information should be provided only on a need-to-know basis to individuals or organizations that use the information to provide treatment, obtain payment, or perform other related health care operations. This includes all patient information regardless of the format in which it occurs—verbal, written, or electronic.

If, in the course of doing your job, you accidentally see or hear patient information that you do not need to know, remember that this information is confidential and that you are not permitted to repeat it to or share it with others. This is the case even when you no longer work for PMG.

Polaris Medical Group's HIPAA compliance officer has developed policies to ensure compliance with the HIPAA Privacy Rule. Every employee is responsible for complying with these policies and protecting patient privacy. You must read and understand the policies related to your job function.

Polaris Medical Group Patient Privacy Guidelines—General

Oral Communication

Oral communication is a common source of confidentiality breaches because others in the office may have the opportunity to overhear a discussion. The following actions should be taken to ensure patient privacy:

- Consider who may overhear your conversation.
- Tell confidential information only to those who have a need to know.
- Speak in an appropriate tone of voice.
- Move the discussion to an area where others will not be able to hear.

If you overhear others discussing confidential information:

- Let them know they can be overheard.
- Keep the information to yourself.

Physical Security

Simple measures can be taken to keep an unauthorized person from gaining access to information:

- Accompany visitors and repair/maintenance personnel to and from their destinations.
- Question individuals whom you do not recognize if they are near areas that contain confidential information.
- Lock all file cabinets, desk drawers, and the like when you walk away.

Using Photocopy Machines

The following guidelines apply to the use of photocopy machines:

- Never leave a photocopier unattended when making copies of confidential information.
- Make sure you have removed all papers from the copy machine before leaving it. Check all areas of the copier—the top of the glass surface as well as all output and input trays.
- Do not allow others to see the information you are copying.

Using Fax Machines

The following guidelines should be followed when operating fax machines:

- Use a cover sheet that shows your contact information and contains a confidentiality disclaimer.

- Confirm the recipient's contact information, including fax and telephone numbers.

- Advise the recipient prior to faxing confidential information, so that he or she may immediately retrieve it from the fax machine.

- Follow up with the recipient to verify that he or she received the fax.

- Immediately remove confidential information from the fax machine.

Disposing of Confidential Information

Never discard paper that contains patient information in a trash can. Doing so makes the information vulnerable to unauthorized personnel. Always shred or dispose of confidential information in a designated container.

Polaris Medical Group Patient Privacy Guidelines— Information Technology

To protect patient privacy and to comply with HIPAA regulations, Polaris Medical Group adopted the following guidelines related to passwords, computer viruses, e-mail messages, printers, the Internet, personal computers, and laptop computers.

Protecting Your Password

You are responsible for all actions performed under your user name and password. Treat your password as you would treat any personal and confidential information by taking measures to keep it confidential. The best way to ensure that your password remains confidential is to use one that is difficult to guess and to change the password as often as every ninety days.

Don't write your password where it can be seen, and don't share your password with anyone, not even the practice manager. If someone asks for your password or if you believe that another person has learned it, report this to the practice manager. If you forget your password or need assistance changing it, contact the practice manager. Remember, you are accountable for any transactions made under your user name and password.

Protecting Your Computer from Computer Viruses

A virus is a computer program that performs unexpected or unauthorized actions. A virus can render a system unavailable and corrupt information contained in a system. To help protect your computer from becoming infected with a virus, never open an unsolicited e-mail attachment or download a file from a source you don't trust. Use antivirus software to scan all e-mail messages and downloads. If you believe that your computer may be infected with a virus, contact the practice manager.

Using Printers

Printers are shared by staff members, which makes it necessary to take measures to protect confidential information when printing:

- Notice the name and location of the printer to which you are sending a file.
- Immediately remove confidential items from the printer output tray.
- Deliver or dispose of confidential information found on a printer.

Using Electronic Mail (E-mail)

Electronic mail (e-mail) is provided for the purpose of conducting PMG business and providing service to our customers. Appropriate use of e-mail can prevent the accidental disclosure of confidential information and the disruption of computer services.

Before communicating directly with a patient through e-mail, you should add the following disclaimer to the bottom of all e-mail communications:

> "By communicating with PMG staff through e-mail, you agree to comply with the e-mail terms and conditions found at www.pmg.com/emailterms. Should you decide that you do not want to comply with these terms, it is your obligation to (1) reply to the PMG staff member with whom you are corresponding, indicating that you do not agree to comply with these terms, and (2) cease further communication with PMG by e-mail."

The following guidelines should be followed when using e-mail:

- Use e-mail only for official PMG business. Don't forward humor, stories, chain letters, or the like.
- Do not send an e-mail message that may be interpreted as disruptive, offensive, or harmful to others.
- When transmitting confidential information, double-check the e-mail addresses of intended recipients.
- Tell the recipient that the information being conveyed is sensitive in nature and should be protected. You can do this by adding the following disclaimer:

> "This e-mail may contain confidential information of Polaris Medical Group. Any unauthorized or improper disclosure, copying, distribution, or use of the contents of this e-mail and attached document(s) is prohibited. The information contained in this e-mail and attached document(s) is intended only for the personal and confidential use of the recipient(s) named above. If you have received this communication in error, please notify the sender immediately by e-mail, and delete the original e-mail and attached document(s)."

- Use available security methods to encrypt messages.

Using Laptop Computers and Personal Digital Assistants (PDAs)

Laptops and personal digital assistants (PDAs) often contain confidential information. Steps must be taken to secure the information contained on these devices.

- Physically secure the device with a locking mechanism.
- Require a password for access.
- Do not leave a laptop or PDA unattended in a public place.

Using Personal Computers

Computers are an access point to confidential information. To protect confidential information:

- *Restrict the view or access of others:* If possible, position your computer screen so that others cannot view it. This will prevent someone from seeing confidential information. Set your screen saver to automatically activate, and hide confidential information when your computer is not in use.

- *Follow appropriate log-on and sign-off procedures:* Never use someone else's user name and password or allow another person to use yours. Prevent others from using your log-on by locking your computer workstation when leaving it unattended. Protect the log-ons of others by always looking away when someone types his or her password.

- *Store files properly:* Do not store confidential information on a local computer workstation unless you are authorized to do so. Instead, store information on your network's shared drive. Delete files that are no longer needed. Secure removable media such as CD-ROMs from unauthorized access by keeping them in a locked drawer or cabinet.

- *Adhere to software installation and removal procedures:* Do not install software that is not approved for use on PMG computer workstations. This includes software downloaded from the Internet, such as screen savers and games, and personal software purchased for home use. PMG must own a valid software license for all software installed on its computers.

Violations of PMG's Patient Privacy Guidelines

The violation of regulations under HIPAA legislation can result in civil and/or criminal penalties. Civil penalties of $100 per violation can be imposed, up to a total of $25,000 in one year. Criminal penalties for wrongfully obtaining or disclosing PHI can range from $50,000 to $250,000 and imprisonment of from one to ten years.

If you feel that a patient's privacy or confidentiality has been violated, report the incident to the HIPAA compliance officer. You may remain anonymous when making the report.

OFFICE VISIT PROCEDURES

When a patient is seen by one of the physicians in the office, employees must follow specific procedures. This section of the PPM describes PMG's office visit procedures.

Receptioning

When patients arrive at the office, the patient services specialist greets them in a friendly manner. If the patient has an appointment, suggest that he or she have a seat and indicate the approximate waiting time to see the physician. If the patient does not have an appointment, ask "How may I help you today?" If the situation is an emergency, calmly escort the patient to an examining room, and immediately alert the practice manager.

If the situation is not an emergency, determine the reason for the visit. Inform the patient that the physician sees patients by appointment only, except in the case of an emergency, but that you will look at the schedule to see whether the patient can be accommodated. Once you have checked the schedule, tell the patient the approximate waiting time.

Gathering Patient Information

The office requires that certain information be on file for each patient of the practice. Basic information is usually obtained over the telephone before the first appointment; more detailed information is gathered when the patient arrives at the office.

Preregistration Information Obtained from New Patients over the Telephone

When a new patient calls to request an appointment, basic information is obtained during the telephone call. This information is used to determine whether the patient is appropriate for PMG (for example, ensuring that the condition is within the physicians' practice areas and determining insurance coverage) and to begin a medical record for the patient. The information must be entered in the computer before the patient can be scheduled for an appointment. The information to be obtained is as follows:

- Name of patient
- Phone number/alternate number

- Address
- Date of birth
- Gender
- Social Security number
- Name of insurance plan
- Reason for call/complaint

A new patient should be asked to fill out a patient information form at the time of the initial office visit. When an established patient comes in for an office visit, ask whether any information has changed since the last visit. If there are any changes, provide the patient with a patient update form to complete. The new information must then be entered in the office computer.

New patients must also be given a copy of the PMG Notice of Privacy Practices and must be asked to sign an Acknowledgment of Receipt of Notice of Privacy Practices form.

Information from Other Sources

When a new patient visits the office, it is often necessary to request patient medical records from the patient's prior physician. The office has a special form, Authorization for Release of Medical Records (see Figure 2-1 on page 52), that must be signed by the patient and then forwarded to the other physician.

Verifying Insurance Coverage

A patient's insurance coverage should be verified before treatment is given, except in emergency situations. Insurance coverage changes under many circumstances, such as when patients change jobs, get divorced, or complete college (in the case of a dependent). Unless patients are seen on a frequent basis (monthly or more often), you should ask the patient whether there has been any change in insurance coverage. In cases in which there have been changes, insurance coverage should be verified before the patient receives treatment.

Guidelines

- If the patient is new or the insurance has changed, photocopy both sides of the insurance identification card (see Figure 2-2 on page 53 for a sample insurance identification card). Insurance identification cards usually indicate the type of coverage, effective date, phone numbers to call, and other data. Verify that the identification number and/or group number matches the number(s) on the patient information form. Also

AUTHORIZATION FOR USE OR DISCLOSURE OF MEDICAL RECORD INFORMATION

Patient Full Name: _____   Medical Record #: _____
Patient Address: _____   Date of Birth: _____
_____   Home Phone: _____
Work Phone: _____

I HEREBY AUTHORIZE POLARIS MEDICAL GROUP (check one):
__ To release my Medical Record information to:
__ To speak about my Medical Record information with:
Other: _____
Name/Facility: _____
Attention: _____
Address: _____
_____

INFORMATION NEEDED   (Be specific, include provider name and dates of treatment, if applicable): _____
_____
_____

(Note: We do not provide copies of records Polaris received from another physician or institution.
Please request those records directly from the original health care provider.)

FOR THE PURPOSE OF: _____
So that we can be sure that your Medical Record information is complete, did you have an appointment with or receive
services from us today? If yes, please indicate with whom: _____

AUTHORIZATION FOR RELEASE OF SENSITIVE OR STATUTORILY PROTECTED INFORMATION.
IMPORTANT : If your Medical Records contains information in any of the following areas and you want this information to
be included in your request, you need to indicate your authorization by initializing next to the corresponding category(ies).
Otherwise, Polaris will not release the following categories, except as required by law.

	YES Release	NO Do not Release	Initials		YES Release	NO Do not Release	Initials
Abortion				AIDS/ARC			
Alcohol Abuse				HIV Tests or related information			
Substance Abuse				Domestic/Sexual Assault			
Mental Health				Sexually Transmitted Disease			

Does your medical record contain any other information that you would like withheld under this release? If yes, please specify; include
provider names and dates, as applicable.   _____
_____

_____
Patient's Signature   Date*

_____
Parent/Legally Recognized Representative Signature**   Date*

_____
Witness   Date

*This Authorization is valid for 90 days (30 days for alcohol/drug abuse treatment) unless you specify otherwise: _____. You may revoke this
Authorization at any time by providing a written statement to the Health Information Management Department, except to the extent that Polaris has
already completed action on it.

**By my signature, I attest that I am the legally recognized representative of the above-mentioned patient in accordance with the following:
_____

The information released pursuant to this Authorization may be redisclosed by the receiving institution or individual to other individuals or organizations
that are not subject to privacy protection laws.

Polaris will not condition treatment or payment on the provision of this Authorization.

FIGURE 2-1   Authorization for Release of Medical Records

check to make sure the policy is in effect as of the date of treatment. A patient may have a card for a policy that is not yet in effect or for one that has terminated.

- Obtain employment information from the patient, especially the length of time with the current employer. Many companies have thirty-, sixty-, or ninety-day waiting periods before insurance benefits are effective.

- Medicaid patients must provide proof of eligibility at the start of every office visit. If a patient's eligibility is not checked, benefits may not be paid to the physician, since Medicaid eligibility changes on a continuing basis.

FIGURE 2-2 Sample Insurance Identification Card

- If a patient has an insurance plan that is not already on file in the office, call the insurance carrier and request a Policy and Procedure Manual. Obtain the following information during the telephone call:

  - Is there a deductible for this plan? If yes, how much? Has the deductible been met for this year?
  - Is there a copayment for this plan? If yes, how much is it?
  - What are the plan benefits for office visits? Outpatient hospitalization? Inpatient hospitalization? Preventive care?
  - What percentage do you reimburse?
  - Which services require preauthorization?

Checking for Preauthorization Requirements

Many payers require preauthorization before they provide coverage for hospital admissions, surgeries, and certain procedures. *Preauthorization* refers to the process of obtaining permission from the payer for a particular service before the care is provided. Since the office works with many different health plans, it is impossible to remember the requirements of each carrier. For this reason, PMG has the Policy and Procedure Manuals of all insurance carriers on file. The requirements of the major health plans, including Medicare and Medicaid, are summarized at the end of this manual (see pages 71-81).

preauthorization
prior approval from an insurance carrier that must be received before a procedure for a patient will be covered under the particular plan

Checking for Referral Requirements

A few managed care plans require referrals from a patient's primary care physician before services provided by another physician will be covered. If the referral is not obtained, the insurance carrier will not pay the claim. The two types of referrals are incoming referrals and outgoing referrals.

Incoming referrals occur when another physician refers a patient to PMG for treatment. In that case, the referring physician will send a referral to PMG, recommending that one of the physicians see the patient. If a patient's insurance plan requires a referral (assuming that one of PMG's physicians is not the patient's primary care provider), you must make sure you have a referral on file for the patient. A referral may be communicated in the form of a letter or a fax or electronically through the computer.

An outgoing referral occurs when one of the physicians at PMG sends a patient to another physician for additional evaluation and treatment. In these instances, if required, PMG sends a referral to the other physician recommending that the patient be seen by that physician. The health plan information pages on pages 71–81 of this manual specify which plans require a patient to obtain a referral.

Concluding the Patient's Visit

Before the patient leaves the office at the conclusion of an office visit, you need to perform certain tasks. If there is a payment or copayment due at this time, inform the patient of the charges, accept the payment, thank the patient, and provide a walkout receipt. If the patient has Medicare or another insurance carrier for which the practice accepts assignment, no payment is due at the time of service. If the physician has indicated that the patient needs a follow-up appointment, schedule the appointment before the patient leaves the office.

Appointments

During the day, many telephone calls coming in to the office are requests for appointments. The physicians do not see patients without appointments.

Scheduling Appointments

Scheduling is sometimes a balance between the clinical needs of patients and the productivity needs of the office. Ideally, patients should not have to wait to see the physician, and the physician should not have to wait for the next patient to arrive. In practice, to ensure that the physician is not kept waiting, multiple patients may be scheduled at the same time. This allows for variations that naturally occur each day—one patient arrives ten minutes early, another arrives fifteen minutes late.

Patient Flow

All patients are scheduled according to their medical complaints. All new or established patients who require lab work, the completion of insurance forms, or the like are asked to report fifteen minutes before they are scheduled to see the physician so that the procedures or paperwork will be completed prior to the appointment time. When scheduling a patient, suggest several available time slots, and allow the patient to choose the one that is most convenient.

If patients are worked into the daily schedule, inform them that they may have to wait a little longer than usual since they were not scheduled in advance. Informed patients are less likely to complain. If it is not an emergency, ask the patient to consider an appointment for another day.

In addition to patient appointments, the following activities are entered on a physician's appointment schedule:

- Regularly scheduled meetings
- Lunch hours
- Hospital rounds
- Days when the physician is scheduled to be out of town
- Days the physician is scheduled to be off
- Surgical schedules
- Other outside activities

Scheduling Allotments

The office has a list of the different levels of office visits for new and established patients and the approximate time needed for each. The time needed is listed in the General tab of the Procedure/Payment/Adjustment dialog box in Medisoft. When a patient calls to request a first appointment, a follow-up appointment, or a comprehensive physical exam, for example, you will know approximately how much time is required. New patients should arrive fifteen minutes before the scheduled appointment to allow time to complete paperwork.

PAYMENT FOR SERVICES

Polaris Medical Group accepts insurance coverage from the major insurance carriers in the region. Both physicians accept assignment for Medicare, Medicaid, and TRICARE patients. Most of the insurance carriers are already entered in the Medisoft database. Occasionally, a new carrier must be added when the practice has established a contract with it.

At a patient's first visit, the patient signs a release form that assigns all insurance benefits to be paid directly to PMG. Should a claim be denied or a portion of the bill not paid by the insurance carrier, the patient may be responsible for the remaining amount. Polaris Medical Group accepts payment in the form of cash, personal check, or credit/debit card.

The Collections Policy

The Polaris Medical Group policy regarding the collection of overdue payments is as follows:

- Patients are responsible for making arrangements to pay for services they receive.
- A patient is required to pay any outstanding balance within thirty days of the date of the service (unless an insurance claim is being resubmitted or appealed).
- If payment is not received within thirty days, a second statement or a notice will be sent reminding the patient that payment is overdue. The patient services specialist may also telephone the patient directly.
- If full payment is not received within sixty days of the date of service, the patient's credit at PMG will be limited until arrangements are made to pay the outstanding balance.
- In some instances, patients may request a monthly payment plan. These requests are considered on a case-by-case basis by the practice manager.
- If full payment is not received within ninety days of the date of service, the patient services specialist sends a collection letter to the patient, requesting immediate payment.
- Questions regarding the practice's collection policy are directed to the practice manager.

The Billing Process

Polaris Medical Group uses a single set of fees for its procedures. The procedure codes and their corresponding fees are listed in the Amounts tab of the Procedure/Payment/Adjustment dialog box in Medisoft. For ease of reference, Polaris Medical Group's current fee schedule is also displayed on page 70 of this manual.

Allowed Amounts

An allowed amount is the amount a given insurance carrier agrees to pay for a given procedure. In some cases, an allowed amount may be the same amount as the provider is charging, as in a fee-for-service plan. In other cases, the allowed amount will be less than the charge amount, as in a managed care plan or a government plan such as Medicare. In Medisoft, the allowed amounts for each procedure by each insurance carrier are stored in the Allowed Amounts tab of the Procedure/Payment/Adjustment dialog box (accessed through the Lists menu). The program uses the allowed amounts in this table to calculate the correct adjustment and to arrive at an estimate of how much the insurance carrier and/or the patient can be expected to pay for a procedure.

Billing Codes, Patient Statements, and Place of Service Codes

The practice uses two billing codes—A and B—to indicate whether patients are insurance patients (Code A) or cash patients (Code B). Patient statements are mailed to patients on a monthly basis. Cash patients are billed at the end of the third and fourth weeks of the month, and insurance patients are billed at the end of the month.

The practice uses the following place of service (POS) codes when entering billing transactions in Medisoft:

Code	Description
11	Office
12	Home
21	Inpatient hospital
22	Outpatient hospital
23	Emergency room—hospital
24	Ambulatory surgical center
25	Birthing center
31	Skilled nursing facility
32	Nursing facility
33	Custodial care facility

Insurance Claims

Insurance claims are generated on a daily basis. Information needed to generate the claims is gathered by the patient services specialist from data found on the encounter forms located in the patients' medical records. The encounter form lists the codes for the most common procedures and diagnoses. After the physician sees the patient, the applicable procedure and diagnosis codes are marked on the encounter form.

The information on the encounter form is then entered in Medisoft. If the patient is receiving treatment for an existing condition, locate the appropriate case in Medisoft. Verify that the diagnosis on the encounter form matches the diagnosis in the Medisoft case. If they match, go to the Transaction Entry dialog box, locate the appropriate case, and enter the procedure code and charges for the current visit. If the diagnosis is for a new condition, a new case must be created before the procedure code and charges are entered.

Reviewing Linkage and Compliance

Before entering diagnosis and procedure codes, always check the data on the encounter form for errors. Make sure the diagnosis listed and the medical services received are logically connected so that the medical necessity of the charges will be clear to the insurance company.

medical necessity
payment criterion of third-party payers that requires medical treatments to be appropriate for a patient's diagnosis and to be provided in accordance with generally accepted standards of medical practice

Medical necessity refers to provisions set up by third-party payers requiring medical treatments to be appropriate and provided in accordance with generally accepted standards of medical practice. These standards require that the service or procedure:

- Matches the diagnosis
- Is not elective
- Is not experimental
- Has not been performed for the convenience of the patient or the patient's family
- Has been provided at the appropriate level

If the insurance company determines that the criteria have not been met—for example, that the procedure performed does not match or link up with the diagnosis listed for the patient—the company will issue a medical necessity denial and refuse to pay for the procedure.

Billing Guidelines

To ensure that payment for services is received in a timely manner, the patient services specialist must follow these billing guidelines:

- Be familiar with currently used procedure and diagnosis codes; understand how to use the CPT and ICD-9-CM manuals to research information.
- Use Medisoft Advanced Patient Accounting to post charges, payments, and adjustments; generate and submit insurance claims; and generate patient statements.
- Explain the practice's payment for services policy to all patients before services are provided. Discuss insurance coverage as well as patient responsibility.
- Provide clear, easy-to-understand statements that list the date the service was provided, the procedures performed, and the charges for those procedures.
- If a copayment is required at the time of service, collect the copayment before the patient leaves the office.

- If a patient is unable to pay the amount due at the time of service, ask for a commitment to a regular payment plan.

- Mail patient statements on a monthly basis.

- If a patient does not make payment when requested and no payment plan has been discussed, speak to the practice manager about the situation.

- Help patients if they have questions about their bills.

- Follow up on all outstanding patient accounts on a monthly basis. Balances are aged as follows: current (0–30 days), past (31–60 days), past (61–90 days), and past (91 or more days).

- Verify insurance coverage before the patient receives services, including deductibles, copayments, limits, and preauthorization requirements.

- Follow up on all outstanding insurance claims on a weekly basis.

- In the event of an overpayment by an insurance carrier or a patient, notify the company or person in writing, file a copy in the patient's insurance file, and issue a repayment if appropriate.

Review of RAs

When a remittance advice (RA) arrives from an insurance carrier, it is important to compare the information on it with other information in the computer. (See Figure 2-3 for a sample RA.) The RA should be reviewed

```
PROVIDER NUMBER:    200000000 (1)                              MEDICAID                                      RA # 09999999 (3)
MEDICAL (5)                                        REMITTANCE ADVICE AS OF 10-10-10 (2)                          PAGE    2 (4)
RECIPIENT MEDICAID        INTERNAL    SERVICE DATES  P  PROC              BILLED  ALLOWED    CUT/        PAYMENT  ADJUST
  NAME       I.D.         CONTROL      FROM    TO    O  CODE-MOD   QTY    AMOUNT  AMOUNT     BACK        AMOUNT   REASON
                          NUMBER     MMDDYY MMDDYY   S                                                           CODES
  (6)        (7)            (8)         (9)        (10) (11)       (12)    (13)    (14)       (15)        (16)     (17)
------------------------------------------------------------------------------------------------------------------------
KROSS,IMA   09004999 1503279009999   092903 092903 11  99213        1     42.44   24.00     18.44-       24.00  A2
                 PAT ACCT:     KR025
                   (18)              092903 092903 11  85024         1     35.00   11.70     23.30-       11.70  A2
                                     092903 092903 11  82948         1     18.00    1.00     17.00-        1.00  A2
                                     092903 092903 11  83036         1     40.00   13.41     26.59-       13.41  A2
                                     092903 092903 11  80061         1     50.00   18.51     31.49-       18.51  A2
                                       ****CLAIM TOTALS :            5    185.44   68.62    116.82-       68.62
*** REMARK CODES:  N59
      (19)
JONES,MARY  05513849 4403280009898   100103 100103 11  99213        1     45.00   24.00     21.00-       24.00  A2
                 PAT ACCT:     JO398
                   (18)              100103 100103 11  82948         1     18.00    1.00     17.00-        1.00  A2
                                     100103 100103 11  36415         1      4.00     .00      4.00-         .00  125
                                       ****CLAIM TOTALS :            3     67.00   25.00     42.00-       25.00
*** REMARK CODES:  N59    MA66
      (19)
SMITH,JOHN  29030841 1503279006789   100103 100103 11  99213        1     42.44   24.00     18.44-       24.00  A2
                 PAT ACCT:     SM145
                                     100103 100103 11  81003         1     12.00     .00     12.00-         .00  125

                                       ****CLAIM TOTALS :            2     54.44   24.00     30.44-       24.00
*** REMARK CODES:  MA66
      (19)
SMITH,WILL  77889911 1503279000987   100103 100103 11  99213        1     42.00     .00     42.00-         .00  22
      ***REMARK CODES:  MA92
        (19)
CORRECTED PRIORITY PAYER NAME:(20) HEALTHCARE
OTHER CLAIMS RELATED ID:      (21) AA345678
OTHER CLAIMS RELATED ID:      (22) 555495755

****CATEGORY TOTALS :    NUMBER OF CLAIMS =         4     11    117.62                      117.62
      (23)                                                     348.88             231.26-
****PROVIDER TOTALS :    NUMBER OF CLAIMS =         4     11    117.62                      117.62
      (24)                                                     348.88             231.26-

                         SPENDDOWN AMOUNT:      .00
                            (25)
------------------------------------------------------------------------------------------------------------------------
** EARNINGS DATA ***                                                      CURRENT
      (26)               NO. OF CLAIMS PROCESSED                             75
                         DOLLAR AMOUNT PROCESSED                          1,752.71
                         CHECK AMOUNT                                     1,752.71
```

FIGURE 2-3 Sample Remittance Advice

before payments or adjustments are entered in the computer, paying attention to the following items:

- Confirm that the charges for the services in Medisoft are the same as the charges listed on the RA.

- Confirm that the CPT codes listed in Medisoft match the codes on the RA.

- Confirm that the payment for each procedure is in line with the expected payment for that procedure. Depending on the type of insurance plan the patient has, the billed amount and the allowed amount will vary. For instance, if a patient is enrolled in a PPO that has arrangements with Polaris Medical Group for a discounted fee schedule, the billed amount will be more than the allowed amount, since the latter will reflect the discount. The patient services specialist must therefore be familiar with the different payment arrangements for each insurance plan when reviewing RAs.

- If the payment is less than expected, review the claim to make sure correct CPT and ICD-9-CM codes were used. If a coding mistake was made, resubmit the claim. If no coding mistake was found and you believe that the payment is not what it should be, file a request for review with the insurance carrier.

- If there are unpaid or denied claims, review the explanation provided, and resubmit the claim if appropriate.

Patient Billing Disputes

In the course of your employment with PMG, you may encounter patients who question the amount they were charged for services. If a patient disputes the charges, refer to the following guidelines:

- Remain calm and always treat patients with respect. Remember that they are questioning charges and services provided, not you as an individual. In addition, medical billing and insurance claims are complex; patients cannot be expected to be familiar with all aspects of billing.

- Gather and review the documents relevant to the amount in question (such as the encounter form).

- If, after reviewing the documents, you still believe PMG's figures to be correct, explain your reasoning to the patient in a logical, step-by-step manner. If the patient is not satisfied with your explanation, refer the problem to the practice manager. No matter how upset or irate the patient may be, you must remain calm.

- If you find an error on the part of PMG, apologize for the mistake and assure the patient that you will correct it today and provide corrected paperwork.

DAILY REPORTS

At the end of each day, several reports are generated that provide valuable information to the practice. These include the patient day sheet and the procedure day sheet. The patient day sheet (see Figure 2-4) provides a summary of patient activity on a given day. It lists the procedures for the day, grouped by patient, in alphabetical order by chart number. Besides listing procedures performed for a patient or group of patients, it lists charges, receipts, adjustments, and balances for the patient or group of patients; and it displays a summary of a practice's charges, payments, and adjustments.

Polaris Medical Group
Patient Day Sheet
6/25/2010 - 6/25/2010

Entry	Date	Document	POS	Description	Provider	Code	Modifier	Amount
BROWNWI0		**William A Brown**						
418	6/25/2010	1006250000	11		1	99212		54.00
		Patient's Charges		Patient's Receipts	Adjustments		Patient Balance	
		$54.00		$0.00	$0.00		$288.60	
CONNODA0		**Daniel Connolly**						
413	6/25/2010	1006250000	11		2	99212		54.00
		Patient's Charges		Patient's Receipts	Adjustments		Patient Balance	
		$54.00		$0.00	$0.00		$457.00	
DAIUTAN0		**Angelo X Daiute**						
419	6/25/2010	1006170000		#0347914 Standard Health Care,	1	PAYSTAND		-180.00
420	6/25/2010	1006170000		Adjustment	1	ADJSTAND		-53.00
421	6/25/2010	1006170000		#0347914 Standard Health Care,	1	PAYSTAND		-17.00
422	6/25/2010	1006170000		Adjustment	1	ADJSTAND		-5.00
423	6/25/2010	1006170000		#0347914 Standard Health Care,	1	PAYSTAND		-70.00
424	6/25/2010	1006170000		Adjustment	1	ADJSTAND		-14.00
425	6/25/2010	1006170000		#0347914 Standard Health Care,	1	PAYSTAND		-120.00
426	6/25/2010	1006170000		Adjustment	1	ADJSTAND		-23.00
427	6/25/2010	1006170000		#0347914 Standard Health Care,	1	PAYSTAND		-2.00
428	6/25/2010	1006170000		Adjustment	1	ADJSTAND		-5.00
		Patient's Charges		Patient's Receipts	Adjustments		Patient Balance	
		$0.00		-$389.00	-$100.00		$0.00	
HIROSYO0		**Yomo C Hirosha**						
414	6/25/2010	1006250000	23		2	99283		150.00
		Patient's Charges		Patient's Receipts	Adjustments		Patient Balance	
		$150.00		$0.00	$0.00		$529.00	
KADAREU0		**Eugene S Kadar**						
408	6/25/2010	1006250000	11		1	99202		88.00
409	6/25/2010	1006250000	11		1	COPAYCIGNA		-18.00
		Patient's Charges		Patient's Receipts	Adjustments		Patient Balance	
		$88.00		-$18.00	$0.00		$70.00	
NISINWI0		**William R Nisinson**						
410	6/25/2010	1006250000	11		2	99202		88.00
411	6/25/2010	1006250000	11		2	29515		114.00
412	6/25/2010	1006250000	11		2	73610		113.00
		Patient's Charges		Patient's Receipts	Adjustments		Patient Balance	
		$315.00		$0.00	$0.00		$315.00	
RENNAMA0		**Marilyn K Rennagel**						
415	6/25/2010	1006250000	11		1	99213		72.00
416	6/25/2010	1006250000	11		1	81000		22.00
417	6/25/2010	1006250000	11		1	82948		18.00
		Patient's Charges		Patient's Receipts	Adjustments		Patient Balance	
		$112.00		$0.00	$0.00		$112.00	

FIGURE 2-4 Patient Day Sheet

Polaris Medical Group
Patient Day Sheet
6/25/2010 - 6/25/2010

Entry	Date	Document	POS	Description	Provider	Code	Modifier	Amount
SZINOMA0		**Martin G Szinovacz**						
406	6/25/2010	1006250000	11		1	99213		72.00
407	6/25/2010	1006250000	11		1	COPAYSTAND		-15.00

Patient's Charges	Patient's Receipts	Adjustments	Patient Balance
$72.00	-$15.00	$0.00	$57.00

Polaris Medical Group
Patient Day Sheet
6/25/2010 - 6/25/2010

Total # Patients	8
Total # Procedures	11
Total Procedure Charges	$845.00
Total Product Charges	$0.00
Total Inside Lab Charges	$0.00
Total Outside Lab Charges	$0.00
Total Billing Charges	$0.00
Total Tax Charges	$0.00
Total Charges	$845.00
Total Insurance Payments	-$389.00
Total Cash Copayments	$0.00
Total Check Copayments	-$33.00
Total Credit Card Copayments	$0.00
Total Patient Cash Payments	$0.00
Total Patient Check Payments	$0.00
Total Credit Card Payments	$0.00
Total Receipts	-$422.00
Total Credit Adjustments	$0.00
Total Debit Adjustments	$0.00
Total Insurance Debit Adjustments	$0.00
Total Insurance Credit Adjustments	-$100.00
Total Insurance Withholds	$0.00
Total Adjustments	-$100.00
Net Effect on Accounts Receivable	$323.00

Practice Totals

Total # Procedures	119
Total Charges	$9,828.00
Total Payments	-$1,705.60
Total Adjustments	-$439.00
Accounts Receivable	$7,683.40

FIGURE 2-4 Continued

The procedure day sheet (see Figure 2-5) lists all procedures performed on a particular day and gives the dates, patients, document numbers, places of service, debits, and credits relating to these procedures. Procedures are listed in numerical order.

Polaris Medical Group
Procedure Code Day Sheet
6/25/2010 - 6/25/2010

Entry	Date	Chart	Name	Document	POS	Debits	Credits
29515		**Splint, short leg**					
411	6/25/2010	NISINWI0	Nisinson, William R	1006250000	11	114.00	
		Total of 29515		Quantity:	1	$114.00	$0.00
73610		**Radiology, ankle, complete**					
412	6/25/2010	NISINWI0	Nisinson, William R	1006250000	11	113.00	
		Total of 73610		Quantity:	1	$113.00	$0.00
81000		**Urinalysis, complete, w/microscope**					
416	6/25/2010	RENNAMA0	Rennagel, Marilyn K	1006250000	11	22.00	
		Total of 81000		Quantity:	1	$22.00	$0.00
82948		**Glucose, blood, reagent**					
417	6/25/2010	RENNAMA0	Rennagel, Marilyn K	1006250000	11	18.00	
		Total of 82948		Quantity:	1	$18.00	$0.00
99202		**OV, NP, Low**					
408	6/25/2010	KADAREU0	Kadar, Eugene S	1006250000	11	88.00	
410	6/25/2010	NISINWI0	Nisinson, William R	1006250000	11	88.00	
		Total of 99202		Quantity:	2	$176.00	$0.00
99212		**OV, EP, Low**					
413	6/25/2010	CONNODA0	Connolly, Daniel	1006250000	11	54.00	
418	6/25/2010	BROWNWI0	Brown, William A	1006250000	11	54.00	
		Total of 99212		Quantity:	2	$108.00	$0.00
99213		**OV, EP, Detailed**					
406	6/25/2010	SZINOMA0	Szinovacz, Martin G	1006250000	11	72.00	
415	6/25/2010	RENNAMA0	Rennagel, Marilyn K	1006250000	11	72.00	
		Total of 99213		Quantity:	2	$144.00	$0.00
99283		**ER visit, Detailed**					
414	6/25/2010	HIROSYO0	Hirosha, Yomo C	1006250000	23	150.00	
		Total of 99283		Quantity:	1	$150.00	$0.00
ADJSTAND		**Standard Health Care Adjustment**					
420	6/25/2010	DAIUTAN0	Daiute, Angelo X	1006170000			-53.00
422	6/25/2010	DAIUTAN0	Daiute, Angelo X	1006170000			-5.00
424	6/25/2010	DAIUTAN0	Daiute, Angelo X	1006170000			-14.00
426	6/25/2010	DAIUTAN0	Daiute, Angelo X	1006170000			-23.00
428	6/25/2010	DAIUTAN0	Daiute, Angelo X	1006170000			-5.00
		Total of ADJSTAND		Quantity:	5	$0.00	-$100.00
COPAYCIGNA		**CIGNA Copayment**					
409	6/25/2010	KADAREU0	Kadar, Eugene S	1006250000	11		-18.00

FIGURE 2-5 Procedure Day Sheet

Procedure Code Day Sheet

6/25/2010 - 6/25/2010

Entry	Date	Chart	Name	Document	POS	Debits	Credits
		Total of	COPAYCIGNA	Quantity:	1	$0.00	-$18.00
COPAYSTAND		**Standard Health Care Copayment**					
407	6/25/2010	SZINOMA0	Szinovacz, Martin G	1006250000	11		-15.00
		Total of	COPAYSTAND	Quantity:	1	$0.00	-$15.00
PAYSTAND		**Standard Health Care Payment**					
419	6/25/2010	DAIUTAN0	Daiute, Angelo X	1006170000			-180.00
421	6/25/2010	DAIUTAN0	Daiute, Angelo X	1006170000			-17.00
423	6/25/2010	DAIUTAN0	Daiute, Angelo X	1006170000			-70.00
425	6/25/2010	DAIUTAN0	Daiute, Angelo X	1006170000			-120.00
427	6/25/2010	DAIUTAN0	Daiute, Angelo X	1006170000			-2.00
		Total of	PAYSTAND	Quantity:	5	$0.00	-$389.00
				Total of Codes:		$845.00	-$522.00
				Balance:		$323.00	

Practice Totals

Total # Procedures	119
Total Charges	$9,828.00
Total Payments	-$1,705.60
Total Adjustments	-$439.00
Accounts Receivable	$7,683.40

FIGURE 2-5 Continued

GUIDELINES FOR MEDICARE, MEDICAID, AND WORKERS' COMPENSATION

Some patients of PMG are insured by federal government programs such as Medicare and Medicaid. Individuals who are injured while on the job are covered by government workers' compensation programs. This section provides an overview of these different programs.

Medicare

Medicare is the federal government's insurance program for individuals age sixty-five or older. Some individuals with disabilities and end-stage renal disease (ESRD) also receive Medicare benefits.

Medicare consists of two major parts, Part A and Part B. Part A covers inpatient hospital services, nursing home care, home health care, and hospice care. People who are eligible for Social Security benefits are automatically enrolled in Medicare Part A. No payments or insurance premiums are required. Those not eligible for Social Security benefits may enroll in Part A if they pay premiums.

Medicare Part B is optional. It helps pay for physician services, outpatient hospital services, durable medical equipment, and other services and supplies. Individuals who choose to enroll in Part B pay monthly premiums, coinsurance, and annual deductibles. Polaris Medical Group files Medicare Part B claims with Medicare for physician services, even physician services that are performed in a hospital. For some patients, Medicare is the secondary insurance carrier. In these cases, the primary insurance carrier is billed first, and then any remaining unpaid amount is billed to Medicare.

In 2006, Medicare began a prescription drug coverage program, known as Medicare Part D, to help beneficiaries pay for the medications they need. This help is available to all individuals with Medicare, although the program offers extra help to those most in need. Enrollment is voluntary; to receive help in paying for prescription drugs, beneficiaries must elect to enroll in the Medicare Part D program. An enrollee must also pay a premium for the coverage.

Medically Unnecessary Services

Services that the Medicare program does not consider generally medically necessary are not covered unless certain conditions are met, such as the relation of the procedure, treatment, or service to the diagnoses. For example, a vitamin B_{12} injection is a covered service only for patients with certain diagnoses, such as pernicious anemia.

If a physician believes that a procedure will not be covered by Medicare because it will be deemed not reasonable and necessary, the patient must be notified before the treatment begins. PMG uses a standard *advance beneficiary notice of noncoverage (ABN)* in these cases (see Figure 2-6 on page 66). The ABN form, which can be downloaded from the Centers for Medicare and Medicaid Services (CMS) website, is designed to:

- Identify the service or item that Medicare is unlikely to pay for
- State the reason Medicare is unlikely to pay
- Estimate how much the service or item will cost the beneficiary if Medicare does not pay

Excluded Services

Some services are not covered under Medicare policies. Excluded services are those that are not covered under any circumstances, such as routine physical examinations and many screening tests. These services change each year. Participating providers, such as those at Polaris Medical Group, may bill patients for services that are not covered by the Medicare program. Giving a

(A) Notifier(s):	
(B) Patient Name:	(C) Identification Number:

ADVANCE BENEFICIARY NOTICE OF NONCOVERAGE (ABN)

<u>NOTE</u>: If Medicare doesn't pay for (D)_____ below, you may have to pay.

Medicare does not pay for everything, even some care that you or your health care provider have good reason to think you need. We expect Medicare may not pay for the (D)_____ below.

(D)_____	(E) Reason Medicare May Not Pay:	(F) Estimated Cost:

WHAT YOU NEED TO DO NOW:

- Read this notice, so you can make an informed decision about your care.
- Ask us any questions that you may have after you finish reading.
- Choose an option below about whether to receive the (D)_____ listed above.
  - **Note:** If you choose Option 1 or 2, we may help you to use any other insurance that you might have, but Medicare cannot require us to do this.

(G) OPTIONS:	Check only one box. We cannot choose a box for you.

❑ **OPTION 1.** I want the (D)_____ listed above. You may ask to be paid now, but I also want Medicare billed for an official decision on payment, which is sent to me on a Medicare Summary Notice (MSN). I understand that if Medicare doesn't pay, I am responsible for payment, but **I can appeal to Medicare** by following the directions on the MSN. If Medicare does pay, you will refund any payments I made to you, less co-pays or deductibles.

❑ **OPTION 2.** I want the (D)_____ listed above, but do not bill Medicare. You may ask to be paid now as I am responsible for payment. **I cannot appeal if Medicare is not billed.**

❑ **OPTION 3.** I don't want the (D)_____ listed above. I understand with this choice I am **not** responsible for payment, and **I cannot appeal to see if Medicare would pay.**

(H) Additional Information:

This notice gives our opinion, not an official Medicare decision. If you have other questions on this notice or Medicare billing, call **1-800-MEDICARE** (1-800-633-4227/**TTY**: 1-877-486-2048). Signing below means that you have received and understand this notice. You also receive a copy.

(I) Signature:	(J) Date:

According to the Paperwork Reduction Act of 1995, no persons are required to respond to a collection of information unless it displays a valid OMB control number. The valid OMB control number for this information collection is 0938-0566. The time required to complete this information collection is estimated to average 7 minutes per response, including the time to review instructions, search existing data resources, gather the data needed, and complete and review the information collection. If you have comments concerning the accuracy of the time estimate or suggestions for improving this form, please write to: CMS, 7500 Security Boulevard, Attn: PRA Reports Clearance Officer, Baltimore, Maryland 21244-1850.

Form CMS-R-131 (03/08)	Form Approved OMB No. 0938-0566

FIGURE 2-6 Advance Beneficiary Notice of Noncoverage (ABN)

patient written notification that Medicare will not pay for a service before providing it is a good policy, although it is not required. When patients are notified ahead of time, they understand their financial responsibility to pay for the service. The ABN form may be used for this type of voluntary notification. In this case, the purpose of the ABN is to advise beneficiaries, before they receive services that are not Medicare benefits, that Medicare will not pay for them and to provide beneficiaries with an estimate of how much they may have to pay.

Medigap Insurance

Many Medicare patients purchase supplemental insurance plans known as *Medigap insurance*. Since Medicare does not cover all medical expenses, Medigap insurance plans literally fill in the gaps in Medicare coverage. Medigap plans are regulated by federal and state laws. Most states have adopted the ten standard Medigap benefit plans that can be sold to individuals living in that state.

Some Medigap plans pay the patient's deductible and coinsurance. If a patient has a Medigap plan, it is the secondary payer; Medicare is the primary payer. The claim is filed with Medicare first. Then, in many cases, the claim is automatically sent from Medicare to the secondary payer (this information is noted on the RA). If the claim is not automatically forwarded to the secondary payer, the office must submit the secondary claim.

Medicare Managed Care Plans

Some Medicare patients choose to enroll in a managed care plan. Doing so eliminates the need for a Medigap policy. Medicare managed care plans, also known as Medicare Part C, often provide services not covered under Medicare, such as coverage for an annual routine checkup, at a small cost or no cost at all. However, there are drawbacks to Medicare managed care plans. Under most policies, services must be provided by a specific network of physicians, hospitals, and facilities.

All Medicare managed care plans must provide beneficiaries with coverage for Medicare Parts A and B, assuming that the beneficiary is covered by both parts. In addition to standard Medicare benefits, many managed care members do not have to pay deductibles or coinsurance. In addition, they may have policies that do not limit the number of days of medically necessary hospital stays. In contrast, Medicare Part A inpatient hospital care is paid during the first sixty days less any unmet amount of the annual deductible. After sixty days, the patient is responsible for paying a portion of the daily charges. Other benefits of many managed care plans include low-cost or no-cost preventive care, such as physical examinations and inoculations, and coverage for services such as prescription drugs, eyeglasses, hearing aids, dental care, and more.

Medicare pays the managed care plan a monthly premium to cover the services patients receive. Most plans charge policyholders monthly premiums, although some have no monthly premiums. In addition, many Medicare managed care plans require patients to pay small copayments at the time of each office visit. These copayments are usually between $10 and $25. Other than the monthly premiums and the copayments, there are typically no other

> **Medigap insurance** an insurance plan offered by a federally approved private insurance carrier that is designed to supplement Medicare coverage

charges, regardless of how many times the patient sees the physician or how many days he or she is in the hospital.

The following guidelines must be adhered to when providing care to a Medicare patient:

- Since PMG's physicians accept assignment for Medicare, the office must accept the amount allowed by Medicare as payment in full for services provided.

- The office is responsible for filing the insurance claims for all Medicare patients.

- If the annual deductible has not been met, the office can collect the charge for the service (up to the amount of the deductible that has not been met) at the time of service. For example, if the unmet deductible is $40 and the allowable amount for today's service is $30, the amount of the service ($30) can be collected from the patient. (This does not apply if the patient is covered by a Medicare managed care plan.)

- If the patient has a Medicare managed care plan with a copayment provision, collect the copayment at the time of the office visit.

- If the office has reason to believe that a service may not be covered by Medicare, the patient can be asked to sign an ABN form.

Medicaid

Medicaid provides coverage for physician services, laboratory and X-ray services, prescription drugs, hospital services, skilled nursing and home health services, family planning, and periodic checkups and treatment for children. Medicaid-participating providers must accept Medicaid pricing for services. Typically, Medicaid recipients are individuals with low incomes who have children, are over age sixty-five, are blind, or have permanent disabilities. Medicaid eligibility varies on a month-to-month basis if the individual's income fluctuates. For this reason, it is essential to confirm a patient's eligibility at every office visit. A patient who was eligible for Medicaid last month may not be eligible this month.

If a patient who is eligible for Medicaid has additional health care coverage through an insurance plan or another governmental program such as Medicare (known as "Medi-Medi"), Medicaid is the secondary payer. File the insurance claim with the other carrier first, and then file for Medicaid benefits after receiving the RA from the primary carrier.

Workers' Compensation

When an individual is accidentally injured while performing his or her job or a job-related duty or becomes ill due to the employment environment, government plans called **workers' compensation insurance** pay for medical services. These plans also provide benefits for lost wages and permanent disabilities. When a patient is covered by workers' compensation insurance, other insurance plans such as long-term disability do not cover the charges until all workers' compensation benefits are exhausted.

Medical information about a patient who is being treated under workers' compensation insurance must be recorded in a separate case in Medisoft. In addition, a separate release form for the workers' compensation claim should be filed. At PMG, workers' compensation claims are submitted to Blue Cross and Blue Shield of Ohio.

workers' compensation insurance the government plan that covers medical care and other benefits for employees who suffer accidental injury or who become ill as a result of employment

POLARIS MEDICAL GROUP
Fee Schedule

OFFICE VISITS - SYMPTOMATIC

NEW
99201	OF-New Patient Minimal	66
99202	OF-New Patient Low	88
99203	OF-New Patient Detailed	120
99204	OF-New Patient Moderate	178
99205	OF-New Patient High	229

ESTABLISHED
99211	OF-Est. Patient Minimal	36
99212	OF-Est. Patient Low	54
99213	OF-Est. Patient Detailed	72
99214	OF-Est. Patient Moderate	105
99215	OF-Est. Patient High	163

PREVENTIVE VISITS

NEW
99381	Under 1 Year	181
99382	1 - 4 Years	189
99383	5 - 11 Years	186
99384	12 - 17 Years	231
99385	18 - 39 Years	215
99386	40 - 64 Years	233
99387	65 Years & Up	259

ESTABLISHED
99391	Under 1 Year	143
99392	1 - 4 Years	161
99393	5 - 11 Years	168
99394	12 - 17 Years	194
99395	18 - 39 Years	178
99396	40 - 64 Years	194
99397	65 Years & Up	155

HOSPITAL/NURSING HOME VISITS
99221	Initial hospital care, det.	185
99222	Initial hospital care, comp.	205
99223	Initial hospital care, high	250
99281	ER visit, min.	100
99282	ER visit, low	125
99283	ER visit, det.	150
99284	ER visit, moderate	175
99285	ER visit, high	200
99307	Subseq. nursing facility care, pf.	63

PROCEDURES
10060	Incision/drainage, abcess	117
20610	Aspiration, bursa	112
29505	Splint, long leg	130
29515	Splint, short leg	114
36415	Routine venipuncture	22
45330	Sigmoidoscopy, flex	276
46600	Anoscopy, collection	89
71030	Chest x-ray, complete	153
73610	Radiology, ankle, complete	113
93000	Routine ECG	84
93018	Cardiovascular stress test	202
99070	Supplies and materials	-----

LABORATORY
80050	General health panel	143
81000	Urinalysis, complete	22
82270	Blood, occult, feces screening	19
82607	Vitamin B-12 test	90
82948	Glucose, blood reagent	18
85027	CBC, automated	34
85651	Sedimentation rate test, manual	24
86360	Absolute CD4/CD8 ratio	263
86592	Syphilis test	27
87070	Throat culture	48
87088	Urine culture	42
88150	Cytopathology, cervical or vaginal	35

INJECTIONS
90471	Immunization administration	18
90472	Immunization administration, 2nd	10
90658	Influenza injection, ages >3	28
90702	DT immunization, ages <7	32
90703	Tetanus immunization	29
90707	MMR immunization	90
90722	Therapeutic injection	27
90723	DtaP - HepB - IPV	81
90732	Pneumococcal immunization	38

Standard Health Care, Inc.

PPO

1500 Summit Avenue, Suite 500, Cincinnati, OH 45000

Phone Number	999-555-2900
Precertification Phone Number	999-555-5556
Fax	999-555-8333

CONTACT PERSON

Gloria R. Saniszar

PLAN TYPE

High-Deductible Health Plan (HDHP) that qualifies for use with a Health Savings Account (HSA)

COVERAGE PROVIDED FOR:

Physician Services	Yes
Comprehensive Physical Examinations	Yes
Prescription Drugs	Yes

PRECERTIFICATION REQUIRED FOR:

Office Visits	No
Surgery	Yes
Second Opinions	No
Lab Services	No
Referral to Specialist	No

DEDUCTIBLES/COPAYMENTS

Deductible Amount	$1,000
Copayment Amount	$15.00
Insurance Coverage Percents	100%
	$5,000 maximum annual out-of-pocket cap

MISCELLANEOUS

Accept Assignment	Yes
Number of Days to File Claims	30

Blue Cross and Blue Shield of Ohio
Fee-for-Service Plan

5000 First Street, Worthington, OH 43085

Phone Number 999-555-1414

Precertification Phone Number 999-555-1416

Fax 999-555-1415

CONTACT PERSON
Rosalyn C. Rimbord

PLAN TYPE
Indemnity

COVERAGE PROVIDED FOR:
Physician Services .... Yes

Comprehensive Physical Examinations .... Yes

Prescription Drugs .... Yes

PRECERTIFICATION REQUIRED FOR:
Office Visits .... No

Surgery .... Yes

Second Opinions .... No

Lab Services .... No

Referral to Specialist .... No

DEDUCTIBLES/COPAYMENTS
Deductible Amount $500

Insurance Coverage Percents .... Carrier 70%; policyholder 30%

.... $2,000 maximum annual coinsurance cap

MISCELLANEOUS
Accept Assignment .... Yes

Number of Days to File Claims 30

TRICARE
HMO

PO Box 1000, Columbus, OH 43214

Phone Number 999-555-0303

Precertification Phone Number 999-555-0304

Fax 999-555-0305

CONTACT PERSON
Lt. Regina Cotswold

PLAN TYPE
HMO

COVERAGE PROVIDED FOR:

Physician Services .... Yes

Comprehensive Physical Examinations .... Yes

Prescription Drugs .... Yes

PRECERTIFICATION REQUIRED FOR:

Office Visits .... No

Surgery .... Yes

Second Opinions .... No

Lab Services .... No

Referral to Specialist .... No

DEDUCTIBLES/COPAYMENTS

Copayment Amount $10.00

Insurance Coverage Percents 100%

MISCELLANEOUS

Accept Assignment .... Yes

Number of Days to File Claims 30

Columbus Medical Care
PPO

3000 Arkady Street, Columbus, OH 43214

Phone Number 999-555-7777

Precertification Phone Number 999-555-7779

Fax 999-555-7778

CONTACT PERSON

George R. Coranelli

PLAN TYPE

PPO

COVERAGE PROVIDED FOR:

Physician Services .... Yes

Comprehensive Physical Examinations .... Yes

Prescription Drugs .... Yes

PRECERTIFICATION REQUIRED FOR:

Office Visits .... No

Surgery .... Yes

Second Opinions .... No

Lab Services .... No

Referral to Specialist .... No

DEDUCTIBLES/COPAYMENTS

Copayment Amount... $12.00

Insurance Coverage Percents 100%

MISCELLANEOUS

Accept Assignment .... Yes

Number of Days to File Claims 30

HEALTH PLAN INFORMATION PAGE

Cigna Healthplan
HMO

1200 Green Avenue, Cincinnati, OH 45000

Phone Number 999-555-9000

Precertification Phone Number 999-555-9002

Fax 999-555-9001

CONTACT PERSON
Ralph B. Granger

PLAN TYPE
HMO, Capitated

COVERAGE PROVIDED FOR:
Physician Services .... Yes

Comprehensive Physical Examinations .... Yes

Prescription Drugs .... Yes

PRECERTIFICATION REQUIRED FOR:
Office Visits .... No

Surgery .... Yes

Second Opinions .... Yes

Lab Services .... No

Referral to Specialist .... Yes

DEDUCTIBLES/COPAYMENTS
Copayment Amount .... $18.00 (in network)

.... $25.00 (out of network)

Insurance Coverage Percents 100%

MISCELLANEOUS
Accept Assignment .... Yes

Number of Days to File Claims 30

Aetna Health Plans

Ohio HMO—Network

5777 Royal Boulevard, Columbus, OH 43214

Phone Number 999-555-1000

Precertification Phone Number 999-555-1002

Fax 999-555-1003

CONTACT PERSON

Elizabeth Kelley

PLAN TYPE

HMO, Capitated

COVERAGE PROVIDED FOR:

Physician Services .... Yes

Comprehensive Physical Examinations .... Yes

Prescription Drugs .... Yes

PRECERTIFICATION REQUIRED FOR:

Office Visits .... No

Surgery .... Yes

Second Opinions .... Yes

Lab Services .... No

Referral to Specialist .... Yes

DEDUCTIBLES/COPAYMENTS

Copayment Amount $15.00

Insurance Coverage Percents 100%

MISCELLANEOUS

Accept Assignment .... Yes

Number of Days to File Claims 30

Ohio Insurance Company
Fee-for-Service Plan

1600 Galleria Way, Cleveland, OH 44000

Phone Number 999-555-5600

Precertification Phone Number 999-555-5602

Fax 999-555-5601

CONTACT PERSON
Lynn Q. Farrell

PLAN TYPE
Indemnity

COVERAGE PROVIDED FOR:
Physician Services .... Yes

Comprehensive Physical Examinations .... Yes

Prescription Drugs .... Yes

PRECERTIFICATION REQUIRED FOR:
Office Visits .... No

Surgery .... Yes

Second Opinions .... No

Lab Services .... No

Referral to Specialist .... No

DEDUCTIBLES/COPAYMENTS
Deductible Amount $100

Insurance Coverage Percents .... Carrier 90%; policyholder 10%

.... $2,500 maximum annual coinsurance cap

MISCELLANEOUS
Accept Assignment .... Yes

Number of Days to File Claims 30

Nationwide Medicare
HMO

P.O. Box 7000, Columbus, OH 43214

Phone Number 999-555-9000

Precertification Phone Number 999-555-9001

Fax 999-555-9002

CONTACT PERSON

Steve Delaplane

PLAN TYPE

HMO

COVERAGE PROVIDED FOR:

Physician Services .... Yes

Comprehensive Physical Examinations .... No

Prescription Drugs .... Yes*

*In some instances

PRECERTIFICATION REQUIRED FOR:

Office Visits .... No

Surgery .... Yes

Second Opinions .... Yes

Lab Services .... No

Referral to Specialist .... Yes

DEDUCTIBLES/COPAYMENTS

Copayment Amount $5.00

Insurance Coverage Percents 100%

MISCELLANEOUS

Accept Assignment .... Yes

Number of Days to File Claims 30

HEALTH PLAN INFORMATION PAGE

Ohio Department of Human Services
Medicaid

P.O. Box 4000, Columbus, OH 43214

Phone Number 999-555-3050

Precertification Phone Number 999-555-3051

Fax 999-555-3052

CONTACT PERSON
Carrie Repinski

PLAN TYPE
HMO

COVERAGE PROVIDED FOR:

Physician Services .... Yes

Comprehensive Physical Examinations .... No

Prescription Drugs .... Yes

PRECERTIFICATION REQUIRED FOR:

Office Visits .... No

Surgery .... Yes

Second Opinions .... No

Lab Services .... No

Referral to Specialist .... Yes

DEDUCTIBLES/COPAYMENTS

Copayment Amount $8.25

Insurance Coverage Percents 100%

MISCELLANEOUS

Accept Assignment .... Yes

Number of Days to File Claims 30

Blue Cross and Blue Shield of Ohio
Workers' Compensation

5000 First Street, Worthington, OH 43085

Phone Number 999-555-1414

Precertification Phone Number 999-555-1416

Fax 999-555-1415

CONTACT PERSON

Harley Burand

PLAN TYPE

Indemnity

COVERAGE PROVIDED FOR:

Physician Services . . . . Yes

Comprehensive Physical Examinations . . . . No

Prescription Drugs . . . . Yes

PRECERTIFICATION REQUIRED FOR:

Office Visits . . . . No

Surgery . . . . Yes

Second Opinions . . . . No

Lab Services . . . . No

Referral to Specialist . . . . No

DEDUCTIBLES/COPAYMENTS

Insurance Coverage Percents 100%

MISCELLANEOUS

Accept Assignment . . . . Yes

Number of Days to File Claims 30

HEALTH PLAN INFORMATION PAGE

Nationwide Medicare
Parts A and B

P.O. Box 7000, Columbus, OH 43214

Phone Number 999-555-9000

Precertification Phone Number 999-555-9001

Fax 999-555-9002

CONTACT PERSON
Steve Delaplane

PLAN TYPE
Indemnity

COVERAGE PROVIDED FOR:

Physician Services .... Yes

Comprehensive Physical Examinations .... No

Prescription Drugs .... Yes*

*In some instances

PRECERTIFICATION REQUIRED FOR:

Office Visits .... No

Surgery .... No

Second Opinions .... No

Lab Services .... No

Referral to Specialist .... No

DEDUCTIBLES/COPAYMENTS

Deductible Amount $110

Insurance Coverage Percents .... Carrier 80%; policyholder 20%

MISCELLANEOUS

Accept Assignment .... Yes

Number of Days to File Claims 30

For questions 1 through 6, write the letter that corresponds to the correct answer in the space provided.

C   1. When a new patient telephones for an appointment, which of the following types of information is usually not gathered during the phone call?
   a. patient's date of birth
   b. patient's Social Security number
   c. spouse's name
   d. patient's address

C   2. A transaction for a patient seen by a physician in a skilled nursing facility uses the POS (Place of Service) code:
   #57
   a. 11
   b. 21
   c. 31
   d. 33

b   3. Which daily log lists procedures performed, grouped by patient?
   a. practice day sheet
   b. procedure code day sheet
   c. patient day sheet
   d. patient statement

a   4. The Standard Health Care, Inc., PPO health plan covers what percent of allowed services?
   #71
   a. 100 percent
   b. 90 percent
   c. 80 percent
   d. 70 percent

b   5. The policyholder's coinsurance amount for the Blue Cross and Blue Shield of Ohio Fee-for-Service Plan is:
   #72
   a. 20 percent
   b. 30 percent
   c. 25 percent
   d. 75 percent

C   6. The copayment amount for TRICARE is:
   a. $5.00
   b. $8.25
   c. $10.00
   d. $12.00

Indicate whether items 7 through 15 are true or false by writing "T" or "F" in the blank provided.

_T_ #65-66   **7.** A Medicare advance beneficiary notice of noncoverage (ABN) is used for excluded services only.

_T_ #31   **8.** Polaris Medical Group defines a full-time employee as someone who works at least forty hours a week and who has worked more than three months.

#40 _T_   **9.** Absences that have been preapproved by the practice manager are considered excused absences.

#54 _T_   **10.** Polaris Medical Group permits the scheduling of two patients in the same time slot.

#59 _T_   **11.** When an RA arrives, the CPT codes listed should be checked against the CPT codes entered in Medisoft.

_F_   **12.** Telephone calls from patients concerning billing inquiries should be routed to the practice manager.

_T_   **13.** Information heard, seen, or read about a patient is considered confidential and should not be repeated to anyone, including members of the patient's family.

#65 _F_   **14.** Medicare Part D, the new prescription drug coverage plan initiated in 2006, does not require a premium and is available to all Medicare enrollees.

#69 _T_   **15.** Workers' compensation insurance covers medical services as well as providing benefits for lost wages and permanent disabilities.

Part 3

On the Job

This section contains the jobs you will complete during your ten-day assignment at Polaris Medical Group (June 14 through June 25, 2010). Jobs are listed by day, and there are typically nine to fourteen jobs to complete for each day. Most days also contain Medisoft Training Topics. Each Training Topic describes a specific Medisoft feature that is needed to complete the jobs for that day.

While completing the jobs in Part 3, you will be using the source documents located in Part 4. In addition, you will be referring to sections of Part 2, Polaris Medical Group Policy and Procedure Manual, for specific information about insurance carriers, scheduling, billing, and other activities of the practice.

As explained in the Getting Started section of the Preface, the Medisoft Student Data files located at the book's website (www.mhhe.com/casestudies5e) contain all the base information needed to complete Part 3. Information about PMG's providers, established patients, and insurance affiliations is already set up in a working Medisoft database contained in the Student Data files. If you have not already loaded this data, go to the website and do so now. The website explains how to download and install the files on your computer.

Whenever you exit Medisoft, you will be reminded to back up your work. For easy reference, it is a good idea to create a separate backup file for each day of the fourteen-day simulation that follows. See the instructions on Backing Up Data in Medisoft in the Getting Started section of this text (page xi).

Using the Allowed Amounts Feature in Medisoft

Medisoft contains an option for storing allowed amounts for each procedure in its database. An allowed amount is the amount an insurance carrier agrees to pay for a given procedure. In some cases, the insurance carrier's allowed amount for a procedure may be the same amount as the provider's fee, as in an indemnity plan. In other instances, such as in a managed care plan or a Medicare plan, the insurance carrier's allowed amount will be less than the provider's fee, since the provider has agreed to a discounted fee schedule in return for other advantages offered by the plan.

In order to estimate how much the insurance carrier can be expected to pay on a claim and how much the patient will be responsible for, Medisoft needs to know the allowed amount for each procedure. Once the program knows the allowed amount, it is able to calculate the correct insurance adjustment (the difference between the provider's fee and the allowed amount). With both the allowed and adjustment amounts in place, the program estimates who can be expected to pay how much.

Allowed amounts can either be stored in the database at the time each procedure is set up, as in the case of the Polaris Medical Group database in this text/workbook, or they can be entered manually each time a payment is received from an insurance carrier. (Allowed amounts are generally listed on the RA.) In the PMG database, the allowed amounts for all procedures have already been entered in the Allowed Amounts tab of the Procedure/Payment/Adjustment dialog box for you. Figure 3-1 shows an example of the allowed amounts for a given procedure.

Once the allowed amounts table has been filled in, whenever a transaction is entered in the Transaction Entry dialog box, the corresponding Allowed Amount for that carrier is displayed automatically in the Allowed column (see Figure 3-2).

Similarly, when a payment is received from the insurance carrier and is applied to the transactions in the Apply Payment/Adjustments to Charges dialog box, Medisoft displays the allowed amount and corresponding adjustment in the Allowed and Adjustment columns (see Figure 3-3). The patient services specialist can compare the amounts displayed with the amounts on the RA to verify that the payment received is correct.

In general, the Allowed Amounts feature makes the payment verification process easier and more accurate.

Insurance Name	Code	Modifiers	Amount
Aetna Health Plans	6		62.00
BCBS of Ohio - Workers' Comp.	10		72.00
Blue Cross/Blue Shield of Ohio	2		72.00
CIGNA Healthplan	5		62.00
Columbus Medical Care	4		62.00
Nationwide Medicare (HMO)	8		39.00
Nationwide Medicare (Trad)	11		39.00
Ohio Depart. of Human Services	9		39.00
Ohio Insurance Company	7		72.00
Standard Health Care, Inc.	1		62.00
TRICARE	3		39.00

FIGURE 3-1 Allowed Amounts Tab for Procedure 99213

FIGURE 3-2 Transaction Entry Dialog Box with Allowed Amounts Displayed

FIGURE 3-3 Apply Payment/Adjustments to Charges Dialog Box with Allowed and Adjustment Figures Displayed Automatically

Note: In addition to filling in the Allowed Amounts table, in order for Medisoft to calculate the required adjustments automatically, the Calculate Disallowed Adjustment Amounts option must be checked off under the Payment Application tab in Program Options. In the PMG database, this option has already been selected as the default.

Study the Medisoft Training Topic, and complete the jobs listed for today.

MEDISOFT TRAINING TOPIC 1:

Claim Rejection Messages

The Claim Rejection Message List in Medisoft is used to store rejection codes and messages received on EOBs (explanation of benefits) or RAs (remittance advices). Once a rejection message is added to the list, it can be attached to a transaction and, if desired, printed on a patient statement to explain why a claim was rejected.

To add a message to the list, the Claim Rejection Messages option on the Lists menus is selected. The Claim Rejection Message List dialog box appears (see Figure T1-1).

To enter a message, the New button is selected. The Claim Rejection Message dialog box is displayed for entering the rejection code and message (see Figure T1-2).

FIGURE T1-1 Claim Rejection Message List Dialog Box

FIGURE T1-2 Claim Rejection Message Dialog Box

The code and message are taken from the EOB or RA. Examples of claim rejection messages are "These are noncovered services because this is not deemed a medical necessity by the payer" and "Claim denied as patient cannot be identified as our insured." The message can be up to 120 characters long. After the code and message are entered, the Save button is clicked to store the new entry.

Once a rejection message is added to the list, it can be attached to its corresponding transaction while applying the insurance payment through the Deposit List dialog box. After clicking the Apply button, the Apply Payment/Adjustments to Charges dialog box appears. To attach the message to the transaction, the rejection message code is entered in the Rejection field to the far right of the Apply Payment/Adjustments to Charges dialog box (see Figure T1-3).

It is also possible to print rejection messages on patient statements. To do so, a patient statement report must be reformatted so that it prints transaction statement notes. To reformat patient statements, the Medisoft Report Designer program (accessed by selecting the Design Custom Reports and Bills option on the Reports menu) must be used.

FIGURE T1-3 Rejection Field in the Apply Payment/Adjustments to Charges Dialog Box

☑ Job 1

If you have not done so already, read the Polaris Medical Group Policy and Procedure Manual (Part 2).

☑ Job 2

Today is Monday, June 14, 2010. Before beginning, be sure to change the Medisoft Program Date to this date. Then open Office Hours, and print today's schedules for Dr. Crebore and Dr. Mahabir. (You will also have to change the date in Office Hours.)

☑ Job 3

Tip!

Job 3

When you set up a new case, remember to edit the Insurance Coverage Percents by Service Classification boxes at the bottom of the Policy 1 tab in the Case dialog box, as different health plans pay different percentages for covered services. For instance, TRICARE pays for 100 percent of covered services, while Medicare generally pays for 80 percent. Insurance coverage percentages are given for each carrier in the health plan information pages (pages 71–81) in Part 2.

When you first view the Policy 1 tab, if the Insurance Coverage Percents boxes are not visible, use your mouse to extend the length of the dialog box so that the information comes into view.

Tip!

Job 4

The default date in Office Hours is the Windows or Vista System Date. You will need to change the date to enter the appointment.

Mary Anne Kopelman, the wife of Captain Arnold B. Kopelman, U.S. Army, arrives at the office for her appointment with Dr. Crebore. She is a new patient. Mary Anne has been experiencing shortness of breath and fatigue. Dr. Crebore examines Mary Anne and orders blood work.

Mary Anne is covered under her husband's TRICARE insurance policy. Her husband is not a patient at PMG. However, information about him needs to be entered in Medisoft because he is the guarantor for Mary Anne. Using the information on Source Document 1 (SD 1) located in Part 4, create a chart number and enter information about Arnold Kopelman in the Patient/Guarantor dialog box in Medisoft (Name, Address tab and Other Information tab).

Then complete the appropriate boxes in the Patient/Guarantor dialog box for Mary Anne Kopelman, and establish a case for this office visit using SD 1 and SD 2. Note that basic information about Mary Ann was entered at the time she telephoned for an appointment.

When completing the Medicaid and Tricare tab in Mary Anne's Case dialog box, use the following information: Non-Availability Indicator: NA statement not needed; Branch of Service: Army; Sponsor Status: Active; Special Program: leave blank; Sponsor Grade: W2; Effective Dates: 06/01/2010 to 05/31/2011.

Once the case is created, use SD 2 to enter today's diagnosis, procedures, and payment (made with check 1011). Whenever you apply a copayment to the procedure charges, the standard practice at PMG is to apply the copayment to the patient's office visit procedure. In this case, the office visit procedure code is 99202. Print a walkout receipt.

☐ Job 4

Angelo X. Daiute telephones to inquire whether PMG is accepting new patients. He has just moved to Fairview and would like to schedule an appointment for a routine comprehensive physical examination.

Establish Daiute as a patient in Medisoft using the information below. Then use Office Hours to schedule the appointment on June 17 with Dr. Crebore at 10:30 (forty-five minutes). You will create a case for him on the day of the appointment.

> Angelo X. Daiute
> 22 Van Cortland Drive, Apt. 390
> Fairview, OH 43773
> Phone: 999-555-1758
> Date of Birth: 1/5/1970
> Sex: M
> SS#: 756-99-2637
> Employer: COSTINC
> Status: Full-time
> Work Phone: 999-555-4300

☑ Job 5

A Medicare RA with a payment arrives (see SD 3) for Lydia P. Stephanos for her office visit on May 27, 2010. Notice that the RA contains a claim rejection message at the bottom. Before entering and applying the payment, add the rejection code and message to the Claim Rejection Messages list in Medisoft.

Then compare the procedure codes and amounts on the RA with those in the Transaction Entry dialog box in Medisoft. If the codes are correct, enter and apply the payment in Medisoft using the Enter Deposits/Payments option on the Activities menu. When applying the payment ($0.00) for the rejected procedure in the Apply Payment/Adjustments to Charges window, tab over to the Rejection field on the far right of the window to record the corresponding claim rejection code.

Note: When applying a payment to charges in the Apply Payment/Adjustments to Charges dialog box, it is important to press Tab to move through each field of the grid. As you tab across each row, Medisoft calculates and fills in any automatic amounts for you, including allowed amounts and adjustments. Since the Remainder amount in column 4 changes depending on what is displayed in the fields to the right of it, you must tab past the end of the row for the Remainder amount to be accurate.

☑ Job 6

Lydia P. Stephanos has an office visit with Dr. Mahabir for treatment of a cyst. Create a new case for this visit, and use SD 4 to enter the procedures and charges for the new case in Medisoft.

Tip!

Job 6
To create a new case for Lydia Stephanos, use the Copy Case button to make a copy of her existing case. Then edit the Personal tab and the Diagnosis tab.

☑ Job 7

Gregory Kavanaugh has an office visit with Dr. Crebore for the routine monitoring of his CD4/CD8 ratio. While in the office, he tells you that his employer and insurance carrier have changed. He completes a new patient information form (SD 5). Using this form, update his information in Medisoft. Note that his new employer is not in the database and will need to be added.

Also, since Gregory has changed insurance carriers, you must create a new case for today's visit, even though it is a routine office visit for an existing condition for which he has been previously treated. Use the Copy Case button to make a copy of the old case. Then update the employment and insurance information in the Personal and Policy 1 tabs respectively. Refer to the health plan information page for the new insurance carrier for details on insurance coverage percentages. Note that even though Gregory has a new insurance carrier, his deductible has already been met.

After the new case has been created, enter today's procedures and charges using SD 6.

☑ Job 8

Victoria Ferrara, an attorney with a local firm, telephones for an appointment. She needs follow-up care for a wound. Schedule her for a fifteen-minute appointment on June 16 at 2:00.

☑ Job 9

An RA is transmitted from Standard Health Care for Martin Szinovacz's office visit on May 19, 2010 (SD 7). Record the deposit/payment in Medisoft, and apply it to the appropriate transactions.

☑ Job 10

Cynthia Cashell phones the office. Her psoriasis has flared up, and she would like an appointment with Dr. Crebore. Schedule her for a fifteen-minute office visit on June 23 at 10:30.

Tip!

Job 11

Remember to select Dr. Mahabir as the provider in Office Hours before making the new appointment.

☑ Job 11

Dr. Mahabir examines Dan Connolly for his complaint of joint pain in the hips. Create a new case for today's visit. Using SD 8, record the procedure for the visit. Schedule a fifteen-minute follow-up office visit for June 25 at 10:00.

❑ Job 12

Cameron Trotta telephones to reschedule his appointment for his annual checkup. It is currently scheduled for June 15 at 3:00. Move the appointment to 2:00 on June 17.

❑ Job 13

Print a patient day sheet for June 14, 2010. Enter *1/1/2000* in the first Date Created Range box, and *1/1/2015* in the second box. Enter *06/14/2010* in both of the Date From Range boxes. Be sure to click the Show Accounts Receivable Totals option at the end of the report box. *Note:* These instructions must be followed each time a patient day sheet is printed (substituting a different date in the Date From Range boxes.)

A Note on the Date Created Range Boxes in Medisoft Version 14: By default, Medisoft enters the Windows or Vista System Date in both Date Created Range boxes. In earlier versions of Medisoft, it was possible to delete the default entries in the Date Created Range boxes and leave the boxes blank so that all values could be included in the report. In Version 14, the Date Created Range boxes cannot be left blank. Some value must be entered. Therefore, for the purposes of the exercises in this text, whenever an all-inclusive range is required for this field, always enter *1/1/2000* in the first box and *1/1/2015* in the second box. By entering this broad range of dates, you can be certain that the full range of data in the database is included in the report.

❑ Job 14

Create insurance claims for June 14, 2010. In the Create Claims dialog box, enter *06/14/2010* in both Range of Transaction Dates boxes. Change the status of the claims from Ready to Send to Sent. *Note:* These instructions must be followed each time claims are created (substituting a different date).

A Note on Claim Status: If claims were transmitted electronically, the claim status for each claim would automatically change from Ready to Send to Sent once the claims were sent. As it is not possible to actually send electronic claims while working on the jobs in this text/workbook, you will be asked to change the claim status manually from Ready to Send to Sent for the claims you create. To change the status of claims, use the Change Status button in the Claim Management dialog box.

The Sent status in the Claim Management dialog box is required when you create patient statements at the end of the simulation. The program generates remainder statements for patients whose claims have a Sent status. Therefore, if you do not change the status of the claims you create to Sent, you will not be able to generate any remainder statements toward the end.

Name _____ Date _____

Daily Worksheet

▰ WEEK 1
DAY 1

After completing all the jobs for Week 1 Day 1, answer the following questions in the spaces provided.

1. What name is entered in the Policy Holder 1 box in the Policy 1 tab (in the Case folder) for Mary Anne Kopelman?

   _____

   _____

2. What are the total charges for Lydia Stephanos's June 14 office visit?

   _____

   _____

3. How many cases are there for Gregory Kavanaugh? Why?

   _____

   _____

4. What amount of the total charges on May 19 is Martin Szinovacz responsible for?

   _____

   _____

5. Who is Dr. Crebore's first appointment on June 17?

   _____

   _____

6. For Dan Connolly, for what amount of the total charges on June 14 is his secondary insurance carrier responsible?

   _____

   _____

7. What were the total patient check copayments made by patients for June 14?

   _____

   _____

Study the Medisoft Training Topic, and complete the jobs listed for today.

MEDISOFT TRAINING TOPIC 2:

Creating a Patient by Insurance Carrier Report and Exporting It to a PDF File

The Medisoft Reports menu contains a Standard Patient Lists option that can be used to create three convenient patient list reports: Patient by Diagnosis, Patient by Procedure, and Patient by Insurance Carrier. Each report lists patients by a different criteria. The Patient by Insurance Carrier report sorts patients according to their providers or facility and then lists them according to insurance carrier. By clicking the Export Report button in the Data Selection Questions dialog box or in the report preview window, the report can be saved to a PDF file.

To generate a Patient by Insurance Carrier report, open the Reports menu, click Standard Patient Lists, and then click Patient by Insurance Carrier on the submenu that appears (see Figure T2-1).

FIGURE T2-1 Standard Patient Lists Option with Submenu

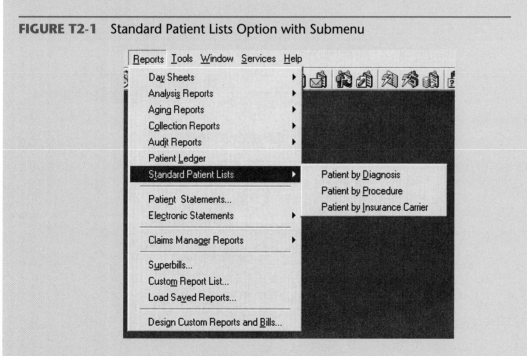

FIGURE T2-2 Export Dialog Box

After clicking the Patient by Insurance Carrier option, a Data Selection Questions dialog box appears, which is used to set parameters for the report. The report can be generated without parameters or it can be created for a range of patients, insurance carriers, providers, facilities, dates, or patient age. Once the parameters are set, click the Preview Report button at the bottom of the dialog box to view the report in the Crystal Report preview window. (Although you can print or export the report from the Data Selection Questions dialog box, it is usually a good idea to preview it first.)

After viewing the report, click the Export Report icon at the top of the preview window to save it to a PDF file. When the Export dialog box appears, click the OK button to accept the default format (PDF) and the default destination (Disk File), as shown in Figure T2-2. (Other format options are available, including Word, Excel, and HTML).

In the Export Options dialog box that appears next, accept the default print range to include all pages in the file. When prompted for a file name, select a folder from the list of folders displayed, enter a file name, and click the Save button. Then exit the preview window. The PDF version of the report can now be viewed or printed in Adobe Reader.

Job 1

Change the Medisoft Program Date to June 15, 2010.

Print today's schedules for Dr. Crebore and Dr. Mahabir. Today is Tuesday, June 15, 2010.

Job 2

Gloria Berkel-Rees telephones for an appointment with Dr. Mahabir. She is due for a three-month checkup on her chronic asthma. Schedule her for a fifteen-minute office visit on June 18 at 2:45.

❏ Job 3

A new patient, Wilma Estephan, arrives for her appointment with Dr. Mahabir. She has complained of pain during urination. Wilma is a Medicare HMO patient. Using SD 9, finish completing the patient information sections of Medisoft for Wilma, and create a case for this visit. Then enter today's transactions using the encounter form found on SD 10. The copayment is paid with check 359. Print a walkout receipt.

❏ Job 4

Dr. Crebore stops by to inform you that she will be out of the office from 3:00 until 5:00 on June 28. Gregory Kavanaugh's 3:00 appointment must be rescheduled. Move the appointment to the same time on June 29, and then enter the break on June 28.

❏ Job 5

David Weatherly, a patient of Dr. Crebore, calls, complaining of difficulty breathing while lying down. He is on hypertensive medications and reports his diastolic blood pressure to be 110. He would like an appointment with Dr. Crebore. Schedule him for a fifteen-minute appointment on June 18 at 10:00.

❏ Job 6

Jimmy LeConey is seen by Dr. Crebore for flu-like symptoms. Jimmy's mother, Ann, reports that Jimmy is no longer covered by her insurance policy; he is now covered by his father's policy. Jimmy's father is not a patient at PMG. Using the information on SD 11, enter Jimmy's father as a guarantor. Then create a new case for Jimmy, and enter the new insurance information. Finally, enter today's transactions using the information found on the encounter form (SD 12).

The insurance deductible has not been met, but first the insurance carrier must be billed. Once the RA is received, the guarantor (Jimmy's father) can be billed for the amount not paid by the carrier.

❏ Job 7

Dr. Mahabir has just finished examining Will Brown. Will complained of rectal bleeding. Dr. Mahabir performed an anoscopy and found external hemorrhoids. Since this is a new condition, you will need to create a new case. Then, using SD 13, enter today's transactions.

Job 8

Roberta Yange-Sang telephones to make a follow-up appointment with Dr. Mahabir for an examination of her laceration. Schedule her for a fifteen-minute appointment on June 18 at 10:45.

Job 9

An RA arrives with payment from Ohio Insurance Company (SD 14). Compare the procedure codes and amounts with those in Medisoft for each patient. If they are correct, use the Enter Deposits/Payments option to enter and apply the payment in Medisoft. While applying the payment in the Apply Payment/Adjustments to Charges dialog box, apply Victoria Ferrara's payment first, and then Gregory Kavanaugh's. When applying Gregory's payment, click the Write Off Balance Now check box at the bottom of the window to write off his remaining balance, which should be less than $10.00. As Gregory has switched insurance carriers, this is the last payment from this carrier for this case. (*Note:* A default code for small balance write-offs, ADJSMALBAL, has already been set up in the PMG database, and the maximum write-off amount is currently set at $10.00.)

After applying Gregory Kavanaugh's payment, open the Transaction Entry window, and locate the adjustment for the small balance write-off in the lower half of the window. Since the program has used the computer's system date for this transaction rather than the Medisoft program date of 06/15/2010, change the date in the Date field to 06/15/2010, and then save the change.

Job 10

George Ahmadian calls to reschedule his appointment that is scheduled for tomorrow at 4:00. Move the appointment to 3:00 on June 17.

Job 11

Dr. Mahabir has finished examining Alan Harcar, who is found to have an upper respiratory infection. Create a new case, enter today's transactions from SD 15, and print a walkout receipt. The copayment is paid with check 1201. Schedule Alan for a forty-five minute appointment for a comprehensive physical examination (CPE) on June 18 at 4:00.

Job 12

Generate a Patient by Insurance Carrier report, and export it to a PDF file. In the Data Selection Questions dialog box, select the Provider option in the Group By field. To include all patients, leave the remaining fields as they are.

Save the PDF file in the folder with your Medisoft backup files, and name it patient_by_ins_list.

☐ Job 13

Print a patient day sheet for June 15, 2010. In the Data Selection Questions dialog box, remember to enter *1/1/2000* and *1/1/2015* in the Date Created Range boxes, and to enter today's date (*6/15/2010*) in both the Date From Range boxes. Click the Show Accounts Receivable Totals option at the bottom of the box.

☐ Job 14

Create insurance claims for June 15, 2010. (Remember to enter *6/15/2010* in both Range of Transaction Dates fields.) Notice how today's claims are added to the previous day's claims in the Claim Management dialog box, bringing the total to eight. Change the status of the new claims from Ready to Send to Sent.

Name _____ Date _____

Daily Worksheet

WEEK 1
DAY 2

After completing all the jobs for Week 1 Day 2, answer the following questions in the spaces provided.

1. What is the amount of the copayment for Wilma Estephan's primary insurance carrier?
   _____ $5 _____

2. Who is listed as the insured in Jimmy LeConey's influenza case?
   Blue cross / blue shield of oHio
   child.

3. What are the total charges for Jimmy LeConey's June 15 office visit?
   _____

4. What procedures were performed during Will Brown's office visit on June 15?
   _____

5. For what amount of the total charges on June 15 is Will Brown responsible?
   _____

6. Who is Dr. Mahabir's first appointment on June 18?
   _____

7. Which of Dr. Crebore's patients have Standard Health Care, Inc., for their insurance carrier?
   _____

8. What are the total insurance payments for June 15?
   _____

9. What is the amount of Alan Harcar's copayment for his June 15 office visit?
   _____

Study the Medisoft Training Topic, and complete the jobs listed for today.

MEDISOFT TRAINING TOPIC 3:

Adding a New Provider

When a new provider joins the medical practice, the provider's name and other data must be added to the provider list database in Medisoft. To add a new provider, select Provider on the Lists menu, and then select Providers on the submenu. The Provider List dialog box is displayed (see Figure T3-1).

The Provider List dialog box lists the current providers in the database. To add a provider, the New button is clicked. The Provider dialog box is displayed. It contains five tabs for storing the new provider's information: Address, Default Pins, Default Group IDs, PINS, and Eligibility (see Figure T3-2 on page 106).

Address Tab   The Address Tab, displayed in Figure T3-2, contains three panels. The top panel contains the Code field, used by the Medisoft program to identify the provider within the program. A provider code can be up to five characters long. If the Code field is left blank, Medisoft assigns a code automatically.

The second panel is used to enter the provider's name, address, and credentials. It also contains fields for the provider's e-mail address and phone numbers.

The third panel is used to record important details such as the provider's Medicare-participating status, license number, and specialty. The Signature on File and Signature Date fields are used if the provider has signed an agreement with Medicare to accept Medicare charges.

FIGURE T3-1   Provider List Dialog Box

FIGURE T3-2 Provider Dialog Box with Five Tabs

FIGURE T3-3 Default Pins Tab in Provider Dialog Box

Default Pins   The Default Pins tab (see Figure T3-3 on page 106) is used to store a range of personal identification numbers (PINS) that the provider may have been assigned from different entities. It contains four panels:

The top panel is used to record the provider's tax ID. Either the provider's Social Security number or federal tax ID number (EIN) must be entered in this field. The radio button to the right of the field indicates which of the two has been entered.

The second panel, labeled PIN, is used to record secondary PINs that may have been assigned to the provider from the major insurance groups, such as Medicare, Medicaid, TRI-CARE, and Blue Cross and Blue Shield. Different providers will have different PINS.

The third panel contains fields for a variety of miscellaneous PINs. Most of the fields in this panel are used to record PINs required for billing specific types of charges or services on electronic claims, including CLIA Number, TAT Number, Hospice Emp, CPO Number, and Mammography Certification. Two more general fields are:

National Identifier: The National Identifier field is used to report the unique ten-digit National Provider Identifier (NPI) assigned to each provider as mandated under HIPAA. The NPI is the provider's primary identifier.

Taxonomy Code: A ten-digit code representing the provider's medical specialty is entered in the Taxonomy Code field. Taxonomy codes are used for administrative purposes on electronic claims.

The last panel in the Default Pins tab contains Extra 1 and Extra 2 fields for recording miscellaneous information as required by the practice.

Default Group IDS   The third tab in the Provider dialog box, Default Group IDS, is used to record secondary group PINS if any have been assigned to this provider by various insurance groups. The fields in this tab are Group Number, Medicare Group ID, Medicaid Group ID, BC/BS Group ID, and Other Group ID—for a group PIN assigned by another type of insurance.

PINs   The PINs tab is available for storing secondary PINs received from specific insurance carriers in the database in table form (see Figure T3-4 on page 108). The table lists each insurance carrier in the database and contains columns for recording a PIN and a Group ID assigned to the provider from that carrier. The table also contains columns for a two-digit qualifier. The qualifier is used to indicate the type of PIN for each PIN or Group ID listed. For example, the qualifier B3 indicates that the PIN has been assigned by a PPO.

Eligibility   The Eligibility tab is used if the new provider participates in online eligibility verification features offered by an insurance carrier. Eligibility verification is used by providers to determine whether their patients are eligible for insurance benefits. In addition, the tab contains a table for storing eligibility enrollment IDs. Some insurance companies

FIGURE T3-4 The PINs Tab in the Provider Dialog Box

require providers to enroll in online eligibility verification by obtaining enrollment IDs. If the provider has been assigned such an ID from a carrier, it is stored in the Eligibility tab.

After the new provider's information is entered in the five tabs of the Provider dialog box, the Save button is pressed to store the information in the database. The new provider is now listed in the Provider List dialog box and can be selected for use elsewhere in the program as needed.

☑ Job 1

Change the Medisoft Program Date to June 16, 2010.

Print today's schedules for Dr. Crebore and Dr. Mahabir. Today is Wednesday, June 16, 2010.

☑ Job 2

Nora McAniff, a new patient who is employed by Argene Interiors on a part-time basis, arrives for her appointment with Dr. Mahabir. She has complained of stomach pain after eating. Nora is a Medicare patient. Enter additional patient information in Medisoft using SD 16. Then enter today's transactions using SD 17, and print a walkout receipt. Nora pays the copayment with check 984.

☑ Job 3

An RA arrives from Blue Cross and Blue Shield of Ohio for Diana O'Keefe (SD 18). Compare the transactions listed on the RA with those in Medisoft. If the RA is correct, enter and apply the payment in Medisoft, using the Enter Deposits/Payments option.

☑ Job 4

Susan Jonas telephones to change the time of her daughter Felidia's June 23 appointment, which is currently scheduled for 11:00. Susan would like to bring Felidia in earlier so that she does not miss half of the school day. Move the appointment to the earliest available time on June 23.

☑ Job 5

Stewart Weintraub calls with an emergency. He has fallen off the ladder in his garage and is afraid he may have broken his arm. Dr. Mahabir meets him in the Emergency Department at St. Mary's Hospital. An X-ray reveals a closed oblique fracture of the left humerus. Dr. Carey, an orthopedic surgeon on staff at St. Mary's Hospital, performs the reduction, and a cast is applied.

Create a new case for the accident, and enter the procedure and diagnosis in Medisoft using SD 19. Note that you will need to fill in the Condition tab since this case is for an accident. Note also that the insurance copayment is not collected, since this is a hospital emergency room visit.

☑ Job 6

Roger Deysenrothe telephones to say that he cannot remember the date and time of his son Floyd's appointment. Locate the appointment in Office Hours, and tell Roger the date and time.

☑ Job 7

Sergeant Georgia Wu telephones to request a follow-up appointment with Dr. Crebore for her daughter Elizabeth. Elizabeth has a mild case of comedonal acne. Schedule a fifteen-minute appointment for June 21 at 4:15.

☑ Job 8

A Medicare RA arrives for George Ahmadian's May 26 office visit (SD 20). Part of the claim has been rejected. Compare the RA with the Medisoft transaction information for this visit. The encounter form for the office visit is SD 21. When you have discovered the problem, correct the transaction. Remember to enter the payment for procedure 82948 in the Enter Deposits/Payments area of Medisoft. When applying the insurance payment, leave the payment box for the corrected transaction blank for now.

☑ Job 9

Victoria Ferrara arrives for her follow-up visit with Dr. Crebore. She has an infected wound that needs to be checked. Using the information on SD 22, enter today's transaction.

☑ Job 10

The practice manager has given you a paper (SD 23) with information on a new provider who is to join the practice next month. You will need to add this initial information to the PMG database. Since Dr. Crebore and Dr. Mahabir are code numbers 1 and 2 in the database, assign code number 3 to the new provider.

☑ Job 11

Flora Torres-Gil telephones to schedule an appointment for her bursitis. Schedule a fifteen-minute office visit on June 22 at 9:45.

☑ Job 12

Print a patient day sheet for June 16, 2010.

☑ Job 13

Create insurance claims for June 16, 2010. Remember to change the status of the claims from Ready to Send to Sent.

Then create a new claim for George Ahmadian's corrected procedure for his visit on May 26, 2010. (In the Create Claims dialog box, enter *5/26/2010* in both Range of Transaction Dates boxes, and select George Ahmadian's chart number in both Chart Numbers boxes.) Change the status of the claim from Ready to Send to Sent.

Daily Worksheet

▰▰ WEEK 1
DAY 3

After completing all the jobs for Week 1 Day 3, answer the following questions in the spaces provided.

1. What is the Medicare amount allowed for the June 16 procedure performed on Nora McAniff?

   _____

   _____

2. Who is Dr. Crebore's next patient after Felidia Jonas on June 23?

   _____

   _____

3. What POS code is used when entering Stewart Weintraub's June 16 transaction? What place of service does it indicate?

   _____

   _____

4. How much did Blue Cross and Blue Shield pay on Diana O'Keefe's account on June 16?

   _____

   _____

5. What is Victoria Ferrara's diagnosis for her office visit on June 16?

   _____

   _____

6. Who is Flora Torres-Gil's provider?

   _____

   _____

7. What were the total insurance and patient payments for June 16?

   _____

   _____

8. What is the balance owed by Diana O'Keefe for her rheumatoid arthritis case?

   _____

   _____

Study the Medisoft Training Topic, and complete the jobs listed for today.

MEDISOFT TRAINING TOPIC 4:

Printing a Patient Face Sheet

Sometimes it is helpful to have a printout of a patient's case information. The Patient Face Sheet report in Medisoft pulls data from several tabs in the patient's Case dialog box into a single-page report. The patient's personal information, such as name, address, employer, date of birth, and so on, is listed at the top of the report. Below that is the case information, which includes fields for the case description, last visit date, referral, guarantor information, diagnoses, and details of the patient's insurance plan(s).

Although it is possible to produce a Patient Face Sheet using the Reports menu, it is more convenient to use the Face Sheet button located in the Case dialog box. After clicking the Face Sheet button, the Print Report Where dialog box appears. (The usual Data Selection Questions dialog box does not display, since the patient and case have already been selected in the Case dialog box.) After an option is selected to preview, print, or export the report, the report is generated.

☑ Job 1

Change the Medisoft Program Date to June 17, 2010.

Print today's schedules for Dr. Crebore and Dr. Mahabir. Today is Thursday, June 17, 2010.

☐ Job 2

Diana O'Keefe calls to schedule an appointment. Schedule her for a fifteen-minute appointment on June 22 at 10:45.

☑ Job 3

An RA arrives with payment from Standard Health Care (SD 24). Compare the procedure codes and amounts with those in Medisoft. If they are correct, enter and apply the payment in Medisoft.

☑ Job 4

Angelo Daiute arrives for an annual exam with Dr. Crebore. Dr. Crebore would like to see Angelo in one week to recheck his blood pressure, which was elevated.

Enter Angelo's personal and insurance information in Medisoft, and then enter today's transactions using SDs 25 and 26. Angelo is a new patient, but his insurance deductible for this year has already been met. He pays the copayment with check 3317.

Schedule Angelo for a fifteen-minute follow-up appointment on June 28 at 1:00.

Job 5

Hector Valaquez telephones the office. He is not currently a patient. His sunburned back is bothering him. He would like to know if the practice is accepting new patients and whether he can come in tomorrow. Establish Hector as a patient in Medisoft using the information below, and then schedule him for a fifteen-minute appointment with Dr. Crebore tomorrow at 9:00. A case will be created for him tomorrow after the appointment.

> Hector M. Valaquez
> 199 Transfer Street
> Highland, OH 45132
> Phone: 999-555-3364
> Date of Birth: 8/15/1982
> Sex: M
> SS#: 459 94 9934

Job 6

The practice manager informs you that she would like case information on Daniel Connolly's chest pain case for billing purposes. Print out a Patient Face Sheet for her to refer to.

Job 7

Dr. Crebore would like Gregory Kavanaugh to be examined by a neurologist to evaluate the seizures he has been experiencing. Check to see whether Gregory's insurance plan requires authorization before a referral to a specialist is made.

Job 8

Rachel Atchely, a resident at Grandview Nursing Home, calls for a follow-up appointment for her cellulitis. Schedule her for a fifteen-minute appointment on June 23 at noon at Grandview. Enter *See at GNH* in the Note box as a reminder that Rachel is to be seen at Grandview Nursing Home.

Job 9

Cameron Trotta arrives for his 2:00 appointment. Dr. Mahabir wants Cameron scheduled for a follow-up visit as he is due for a five-year flexible sigmoidoscopy (45330). Schedule a sixty-minute appointment for June 30 at 10:00. Using SD 27, enter the charges and copayment (check 869), and print a walkout receipt.

Job 10

Seymour Colbs calls. He needs to change his appointment. He is currently scheduled for 4:00 tomorrow. He would like to come in earlier, if possible. Reschedule the appointment for 9:30 tomorrow with Dr. Crebore.

Job 11

George Ahmadian has diabetes mellitus and hypertension. He has been experiencing increasing confusion, agitation, and short-term memory loss over the past two months. He has just been examined by Dr. Mahabir. Using SD 28, create a new case, and enter today's transactions.

Job 12

An RA arrives with payment from Standard Health Care (SD 29). Compare the procedure codes and amounts with those in Medisoft. If they are correct, enter and apply the payment in Medisoft.

Job 13

Print a patient day sheet for June 17, 2010.

Job 14

Create insurance claims for June 17, 2010. Change the status of the claims.

Daily Worksheet

▭ WEEK 1
DAY 4

After completing all the jobs for Week 1 Day 4, answer the following questions in the spaces provided.

1. What is the total amount owed by George Ahmadian for his office visit on June 17, assuming that his insurance carrier pays its portion of the claim?

   _____

   _____

2. What is the name and phone number for the secondary insurance company listed on Daniel Connolly's Patient Face Sheet for his chest pain case?

   _____

   _____

3. What procedure is Cameron Trotta scheduled for on June 30? How much time is scheduled for the appointment?

   _____

   _____

4. What time is Seymour Colbs's appointment on June 18?

   _____

   _____

5. What is George Ahmadian's diagnosis for his June 17 office visit?

   _____

   _____

6. What were the total procedure charges for June 17?

   _____

   _____

7. What were the total insurance payments for June 17?

   _____

   _____

Study the Medisoft Training Topic, and complete the jobs listed for today.

MEDISOFT TRAINING TOPIC 5:

Using Quick Balance

Medisoft's Quick Balance feature simplifies the task of discovering the amount owed on a patient account. This feature can be accessed by pressing the Quick Balance speed button located on the tool bar (see Figure T5-1). If the Quick Balance feature is activated from within the Transaction Entry dialog box or the Patient/Guarantor dialog box, the information will be displayed for the patient who is currently selected. For example, if the Transaction Entry box lists Diana O'Keefe's data, pressing the Quick Balance button will display the balance on her account. A sample Quick Balance dialog box is shown in Figure T5-2.

The dialog box lists all the patients for whom this individual is guarantor. For example, the Quick Balance dialog box for Roger Deysenrothe lists Roger, his wife Mae, and his son Floyd, since Roger is the guarantor on all three accounts. The amount listed as the Guarantor Remainder Total is the amount owed by the guarantor *after* the insurance carrier has paid on the claim. If the insurance carrier has not yet paid, the balance for the account will be zero.

Note that the information can be printed from within the Quick Balance dialog box. In addition, the balance for another patient can be viewed by selecting a different chart number in the Chart field.

FIGURE T5-1 Quick Balance Speed Button on Toolbar

FIGURE T5-2 Quick Balance Dialog Box

☑ Job 1

Change the Medisoft Program Date to June 18, 2010.

Print today's schedules for Dr. Crebore and Dr. Mahabir. Today is Friday, June 18, 2010.

☑ Job 2

Hector Valaquez, a new patient, is examined by Dr. Crebore. Enter patient information about Hector using SD 30, and record today's transactions using SD 31. Hector pays his copayment with check 3231 and needs a walkout receipt.

☑ Job 3

Seymour Colbs arrives for his office visit. Dr. Crebore removes the sutures in Seymour's hand. Enter today's transactions in Medisoft using SD 32. The copayment is paid with check 839. Print a walkout receipt.

☑ Job 4

David Weatherly, a patient of Dr. Crebore who is on hypertensive medication and who is experiencing difficulty breathing, arrives for his office visit. He is examined by Dr. Crebore. Using SD 33, create a new case, and enter the transactions in Medisoft. The copayment is made with check 2312, and a walkout receipt is printed.

☑ Job 5

Victoria Ferrara telephones. She would like to know the balance due on her account. Use the Quick Balance shortcut key to determine the amount. Compare this amount with the information displayed in the Transaction Entry dialog box. Remember that the Quick Balance dialog box displays the amount owed *after* the insurance carrier has paid a claim. In Victoria's case, notice that only the first claim has been paid.

☑ Job 6

Myrna Beedon telephones. She reports that she has felt extremely tired for the past few days. She would like to see Dr. Mahabir. Schedule her for a fifteen-minute appointment on June 21 at 4:00.

☑ Job 7

Mae Deysenrothe calls to reschedule her appointment on June 21 at 10:00 with Dr. Mahabir. Reschedule her for June 23 at 2:15.

❏ Job 8

Review the audit/edit report received for Rachel Atchely's claim (SD 34). Rachel, who resides at the Grandview Nursing Home, is a patient of Dr. Mahabir. Dr. Mahabir's visit on May 26 was for a brief check-up. Identify the error in the procedure code, and edit the transaction using the correct code (99307—Subseq. nursing facility care, pf.).

Then create a new claim for the visit. Remember to enter *5/26/2010* in both Range of Transaction Dates boxes, and to select Rachel Atchely's chart number in both Chart Number boxes. Change the status of the claim from Ready to Send to Sent.

❏ Job 9

Roberta Yange-Sang arrives for an examination of her laceration. Roberta is a Medicaid patient. During the visit, Dr. Mahabir notes that the wound is clear. Roberta is instructed to return in ten days for a recheck.

Enter today's transactions using SD 35 (the copayment is paid with check 240), print a walkout receipt, and schedule Roberta for a fifteen-minute follow-up appointment on June 28 at 10:00.

❏ Job 10

Gloria Berkel-Rees comes in for her three-month checkup with Dr. Mahabir. She has chronic asthma along with hay fever. She also needs drug therapy evaluation. Using SD 36, enter the charges. Note that the charge for procedure code 99070 (Supplies and materials) is set to 0.00 in the database as the amount varies depending on what supplies and materials are ordered. The amount charged for today's encounter is shown on the encounter form. Remember to record this amount in both the Amount and Allowed fields when you enter the transaction.

❏ Job 11

Chantalle Usdan calls the office to schedule a sigmoidoscopy. She has been referred to Dr. Mahabir by her primary care physician, Dr. Rachel Innanni.

Establish Chantalle as a patient in Medisoft using the information below. Schedule her for a sixty-minute appointment on June 23 at 10:00. A case can be created on the day of the visit.

> Chantalle E. Usdan
> 28 Fairview Blvd.
> Columbus, OH 43214

Phone: 999-555-4555

Date of Birth: 2/23/1954

Sex: F

SS#: 234-60-8721

❏ Job 12

Alan Harcar arrives for his comprehensive physical examination. Create a new case, and record today's transactions using SD 37 (the copayment is made with check 1024). Print a walkout receipt. (*Hint*: A MultiLink code is available for help in entering four of the five procedures.)

❏ Job 13

Print a patient day sheet for June 18, 2010.

❏ Job 14

Create insurance claims for June 18, 2010. Change the status of the claims.

Daily Worksheet

WEEK 1
DAY 5

After completing all the jobs for Week 1 Day 5, answer the following questions in the spaces provided.

1. What is Hector Valaquez's primary insurance carrier? How much is his copayment?

_____

_____

2. For his June 18 office visit, for what amount of the charges is Seymour Colbs responsible?

_____

_____

3. What is the diagnosis for David Weatherly's June 18 office visit?

_____

_____

4. How much time is scheduled for Mae Deysenrothe's appointment on June 23?

_____

_____

5. What is the amount Medicaid owes for Roberta Yange-Sang's June 18 office visit?

_____

_____

6. What procedures were performed at Gloria Berkel-Rees's June 18 office visit?

_____

_____

7. What is the diagnosis for Alan Harcar's June 18 office visit?

_____

_____

8. What were the total number of procedures performed on June 18?

_____

_____

End-of-Week-1 Job

Printing a Copayment Report

The Medisoft Reports menu contains an option for printing a copayment report. The report creates an alphabetical listing of all patients who have made copayments and includes the date of each payment as well as the case number, payment code, and amount paid. The amount paid is further broken down into applied and unapplied amounts. A total line at the bottom lists the total copayment amount and total applied and unapplied amounts.

To generate a copayment report, open the Reports menu, click Analysis Reports, and then click Copayment Report on the submenu that appears. The associated Data Selection Questions dialog box that appears is used to set parameters for the report. The report can be generated without parameters, or it can be created for a range of dates, patients, and/or providers. The buttons at the bottom of the Data Selection Questions dialog box are used to preview the report, print it, or export it to another file format, such as PDF, Excel, or Word.

❑ Job 1

Print a copayment report for all patients for the period of June 14 through June 18, 2010.

▰▰ WEEK 2
DAY 1

Study the Medisoft Training Topic, and complete the jobs listed for today.

Entering Prior Authorization Numbers

Sometimes insurance carriers require services to be authorized before they are performed. If preauthorization is not given, the claim will not be paid. Once preauthorization numbers are obtained from the insurance carrier, they are entered in Medisoft. This information is entered in the Prior Authorization Number box, which is found in the Miscellaneous tab of the Case folder (see Figure T7-1 on page 126). From one to fifteen characters can be entered in the Prior Authorization Number box.

FIGURE T7-1 Miscellaneous Tab of Case Folder with Prior Authorization Number Box

☐ Job 1

Change the Medisoft Program Date to June 21, 2010.

Print today's schedules for Dr. Crebore and Dr. Mahabir. Today is Monday, June 21, 2010.

☐ Job 2

There is a message from Myrna Beedon, a Medicare patient of Dr. Mahabir who has a history of congenital heart disease. She was scheduled for a 4:00 appointment today. After you relate the message to Dr. Mahabir, he orders her admitted to St. Mary's Hospital and visits her there. Enter the preauthorization number for Myrna's hospital admission, HA46230, in the appropriate box in the Case folder. Then enter the transactions using SD 38. Note that no copayment is collected since this is a hospital visit.

☐ Job 3

Dan Connolly calls to reschedule the appointment that is currently scheduled for June 25 at 10:00. Change the appointment to 2:45 on the same day.

☑ Job 4

Fran Ferrone is a new patient who has come in for her appointment with Dr. Crebore because of possible bronchitis. Fran is employed by Woodworkers Warehouse in Fairview. The company is not in the Medisoft database of employers, so you will need to add it, using the information on SD 39.

When you call Fran's insurance carrier to verify coverage, you learn that she has met the $500.00 deductible for the year. Complete the Other Information tab in the Patient/Guarantor dialog box for Fran, and set up a case using SD 39. When completing the Policy 1 tab in the Case dialog box, remember to refer to the Health Plan Information Pages in Part 2 to obtain the correct insurance coverage percentages for her plan. Enter today's diagnosis and transactions using the encounter form found on SD 40.

☑ Job 5

Ann LeConey telephones. She needs an appointment with Dr. Mahabir for a recheck of an irritated patch of skin on her arm. Schedule her for a fifteen-minute appointment on June 23 at 4:30.

☐ Internet Activity

Go to the website for Aetna. Look up information on the different types of health plans offered. Explore the member and provider areas of the website.

☑ Job 6

Susan Jonas calls the office to say that her dermatitis has flared up and that she would like an appointment. Schedule her for a fifteen-minute appointment at 4:30 on June 24.

☑ Job 7

Jimmy Hellery is examined by Dr. Mahabir. He has complained of a severe sore throat and fever. Set up a new case. Enter the transactions in Medisoft using SD 41, and print a walkout receipt. The copayment is made with check 1019.

☑ Job 8

Roger Deysenrothe brings his son Floyd in for a tetanus vaccine. Create a new case. Using SD 42, record the transactions in Medisoft, and print a walkout receipt. The copayment is made with check 1117.

☑ Job 9

A remittance advice has arrived from Will Brown's insurance carrier (SD-43). Review the RA, enter the payment, and apply it to Brown's account.

☑ Job 10

Georgia Wu brings her daughter Elizabeth in for an appointment with Dr. Crebore to check Elizabeth's mild case of comedonal acne of the cheeks. Enter the transactions in Medisoft, including the payment (made with check 1202), using SD 44. Print a walkout receipt.

☑ Job 11

Marilyn Rennagel, a patient of Dr. Crebore, calls for an appointment. She needs routine monitoring of her diabetes mellitus and stable coronary artery disease. Schedule her for a fifteen-minute appointment on June 25 at 3:00.

☑ Job 12

Print a patient day sheet for June 21, 2010.

☑ Job 13

Create insurance claims for June 21, 2010. Change the status of the claims.

Name _____ Date _____

Daily Worksheet

▰ WEEK 2
DAY 1

After completing all the jobs for Week 2 Day 1, answer the following questions in the spaces provided.

1. What POS code is entered for Myrna Beedon's transactions on June 21?

   _____

   _____

2. Where is the preauthorization number for Myrna Beedon's hospital admission entered in Medisoft?

   _____

   _____

3. Who has the appointment with Dr. Mahabir before Ann LeConey on June 23?

   _____

   _____

4. What is the amount of the copayment Joan Hellery pays for her son Jimmy's visit on June 21?

   _____

   _____

5. What is Floyd Deysenrothe's diagnosis for his June 21 office visit?

   _____

   _____

6. What is the total amount of copayments made on June 21?

   _____

   _____

7. What are the total procedure charges for June 21?

   _____

   _____

8. What were the total insurance payments for June 21?

   _____

   _____

WEEK 2
DAY 2

Study the Medisoft Training Topics, and complete the jobs listed for today.

Entering Additional Diagnosis Codes

Before a diagnosis code can be selected in the Diagnosis tab of the Case folder, it must be entered in the database. To add a diagnosis code to the database, select Diagnosis Codes from the Lists menu. The Diagnosis List dialog box is displayed. It lists all the diagnosis codes already entered. The codes are listed in numerical order by code number or alphabetically by description, depending on the setting in the Field box at the top of the dialog box.

To add a new diagnosis code, click the New button at the bottom of the dialog box. The Diagnosis: (new) dialog box is displayed (see Figure T8-1). Enter the diagnosis code in the Code 1 box and a description of the diagnosis in the Description box (from one to forty-eight characters can be used). When the code and description have been entered, click the Save button.

FIGURE T8-1   Diagnosis Dialog Box

Adding a New Insurance Carrier

Whenever required, a new insurance carrier can be added to the database. To add a new carrier, select Insurance on the Lists menu, and then select Carriers on the submenu. The Insurance Carrier List dialog box is displayed (see Figure T9-1 on page 132), listing the carriers currently in the database.

To add a new carrier, the New button is clicked. The Insurance Carrier: (new) dialog box is displayed. It contains six tabs for storing the new carrier's information: Address, Options, EDI/Eligibility, Codes, Allowed, and PINs (see Figure T9-2 on page 132).

FIGURE T9-1 Insurance Carrier List Dialog Box

FIGURE T9-2 Insurance Carrier Dialog Box with Six Tabs

Address   The Address tab (shown in Figure T9-2) is divided into three panels. The top panel contains the Code field, used by the Medisoft program to identify the insurance carrier within the program.

The second and third panels contain standard fields for the carrier's name, address, phone, fax, contact person, and practice ID. The practice ID is a number given to the practice by the insurance carrier.

Options   The Options tab contains two panels (see Figure T9-3). The top panel displays fields for identifying the plan name, type, and ID, as well as an option for delaying secondary billing. The Delay Secondary Billing option is used to indicate whether a secondary claim form should be printed at the same time as the primary claim is printed (the default setting), or if the printing should be delayed until an RA is received and a payment or adjustment has been made for the primary carrier. To delay printing, the option is clicked, and a check mark is displayed in the field.

The bottom panel in the Options tab contains various billing options. Several apply to paper claims only:

Patient, Insured, or Physician Signature on File: These fields are used to control what is printed in specific boxes on the CMS-1500 (previously known as HCFA-1500) paper claim form. Options include printing the words *Signature on File* if these fields have been activated in the patient and provider records; printing the party's name (patient, insured, or physician); or leaving the box blank, which is the default setting.

Print PINs on Forms: This field is used on paper claims to record an attending provider's PIN (when the attending provider is other than the usual assigned provider).

Default Billing Method: This field identifies whether claims for this carrier are to be printed on paper or transmitted electronically.

EDI/Eligibility   If the new carrier transmits claim information electronically and/or offers online eligibility verification for checking the status of a patient's insurance eligibility, this

---

FIGURE T9-3   Options Tab

tab is used to select numbers or data connected with such transactions. For example, the EDI Receiver field is for selecting the EDI receiver to which this insurance carrier's claims are sent. For most fields in this tab, the practice's electronic claims manual must be referred to in order to determine whether a number is required.

Codes   The Codes tab is used to select the default codes to be used when entering payments, adjustments, withhold amounts, deductibles, and take backs for the new carrier. Codes are first created in the Procedure/Payment/Adjustment dialog box and then selected as defaults in the Codes tab.

Allowed   The Allowed tab (see Figure T9-4) contains a table for storing the new insurance carrier's allowed amounts for each procedure code in the database. The program uses the allowed amount for each procedure to determine the patient's responsibility.

Amounts may be entered in the table manually, as in the case of the PMG database, or they may be stored by the program automatically—the program calculates the allowed amount based on the amount last paid by the carrier for each procedure. Information entered in this tab also appears simultaneously in the Allowed Amounts tab of the Procedure/Payment/Adjustment dialog box (see Training Topic 13: Entering Additional Procedure Codes and Allowed Amounts). Allowed amounts can be entered through either dialog box.

PINs   The PINs tab is available for storing PINs that the new carrier may assign to the providers in the practice. The information is stored in table form (see Figure T9-5), with columns for recording a PIN and a Group ID for each provider, as well as a two-digit qualifier for each number. The qualifier indicates the PIN type, such as 0B for a state license number. The information in the PINs tab is also available simultaneously in the PINs tab of the Provider dialog box. Information can be entered through either dialog box.

FIGURE T9-4   Allowed Tab

Insurance Carrier: Standard Health Care, Inc.

Code	Provider	Pin	Qualifier	Group ID	Qualifier
1	Crebore, Robin C				
2	Mahabir, Michael P				
3	Sylvia, Serto T				

After information on the new insurance carrier is entered in the six tabs of the Insurance Carrier dialog box, the Save button is clicked. The new carrier is now listed in the Insurance Carrier dialog box and can be selected for use from elsewhere in the program as needed.

❑ Job 1

Change the Medisoft Program Date to June 22, 2010.

Print today's schedules for Dr. Crebore and Dr. Mahabir. Today is Tuesday, June 22, 2010.

❑ Job 2

Martin Szinovacz calls to schedule an appointment to have his blood pressure checked. Schedule him for a fifteen-minute appointment on June 25 at 9:15.

❑ Job 3

The practice manager has just handed you a list of additional diagnosis codes that need to be added to the database (SD 45). Enter the codes in Medisoft.

❑ Job 4

Flora Torres-Gil has an office visit with Dr. Crebore for treatment of the recurrent bursitis in her left shoulder. Enter the transactions in Medisoft using SD 46. Flora pays with check 1309. Print a walkout receipt.

❑ Job 5

Eugene Kadar calls to request an appointment with one of the physicians. He is not currently a patient of the practice. Eugene has recurring sores on his lip.

Establish Eugene as a patient in Medisoft. Then schedule him for a fifteen-minute appointment with Dr. Crebore on June 25 at 10:15. A case will be created on the day of the appointment.

> Eugene S. Kadar
> 8003 Oxford Lane
> Highland, OH 45132
> Phone: 999-555-5858
> Date of Birth: 6/1/77
> Sex: M
> SS#: 499-09-7453

☐ Job 6

Jorge Martinez calls to ask whether he can change the time of his appointment with Dr. Mahabir on June 24. He has a meeting he must attend at work. Locate Jorge's current appointment in Medisoft, and change it to 4:00 on the same day.

☐ Job 7

The new provider who is to join the practice next month has a contract with an insurance carrier not currently in the PMG database. Use the information contained in SDs 47 and 48 to add the new carrier. In the Address tab, use code number 12 for the new carrier, since that is the next number in sequence.

Note: For the purposes of this job, the codes to be selected in the Codes tab have already been created and stored in the Procedure/Payment/Adjustment dialog box for you. For information on creating codes, see Training Topic 13: Entering Additional Procedure Codes and Allowed Amounts.

☐ Job 8

Diana O'Keefe comes in for her sedimentation rate test. Record the transaction using SD 49.

Internet Activity

Go to the website for the Blue Cross and Blue Shield Association. Look up information about the different health plans offered. Explore areas of interest.

☐ Job 9

Print a patient day sheet for June 22, 2010.

☐ Job 10

Create insurance claims for June 22, 2010. Change the status of the claims.

Name _____ Date _____

Daily Worksheet

WEEK 2
DAY 2

After completing all the jobs for Week 2 Day 2, answer the following questions in the spaces provided.

1. What diagnosis code comes right before 794.31, Abnormal ECG?

   _____

   _____

2. What is the charge for the procedure performed on Flora Torres-Gil on June 22?

   _____

   _____

3. Who is scheduled to see Dr. Crebore before Eugene Kadar on June 25?

   _____

   _____

4. What code is used for entering payments from Ohio Maxcare?

   _____

   _____

5. What is the balance on Diana O'Keefe's account as of June 22?

   _____

   _____

6. What is the net effect on accounts receivable for transactions on June 22?

   _____

   _____

7. How many insurance claims were created on June 22?

   _____

   _____

Study the Medisoft Training Topics, and complete the jobs listed for today.

MEDISOFT TRAINING TOPIC 10:

Entering Referrals

Some patients may be referred to the practice by other physicians. These physicians are called referring providers. For insurance billing purposes, these referrals must be recorded in Medisoft. Many managed care plans require patients to be referred by their primary care physician before being treated by another physician. In these situations, if there is no referral, the insurance carrier is not obligated to pay the claim. Often, as part of the referral, a visit authorization number is also required (see Training Topic 11 below).

Provider referrals are entered in the Account tab within the patient's Case folder (see Figure T10-1). The provider referral is entered by selecting the physician from the list of choices in the Referring Provider drop-down list. A provider who is not listed in the Referring Provider drop-down list needs to be added to the database by selecting Referring Providers on the Lists menu and then clicking the New button.

In addition, some practices keep track of other types of referrals, such as the way a new patient found out about the practice. Many physicians like to have a record of referrals so

FIGURE T10-1 Account Tab of the Case Folder

they can review the sources of their referrals. This type of referral can be recorded by selecting the appropriate person or entity in the Referral Source drop-down list, also located in the Account tab (see Figure T10-1 on page 139).

Entering Visit Authorization Numbers

Visit authorization numbers are assigned by managed care insurance carriers, usually when a patient has a referral. In Medisoft, these authorization numbers are entered in the Visit Series Authorization Number box located in the Account tab of the Case folder (see Figure T10-1 on page 139).

Closing Cases

Medical practices have different policies regarding when a case may be closed. Cases are generally closed when (1) the patient is no longer receiving treatment for the condition

FIGURE T12-1 Personal Tab of the Case Folder with Case Closed Box Checked specified in the case and (2) the case has a zero balance. For example, a patient's case for influenza may be closed once the physician indicates that the patient has fully recovered from the condition and when all payments have been received. Cases for chronic conditions, such as diabetes mellitus, may never be closed as long as the individual is a patient of the practice. When an individual is no longer a patient and the account has a zero balance, the case is usually closed.

Cases are closed in Medisoft by clicking the Case Closed box in the Personal tab of the patient's Case folder (see Figure T12-1). A check mark in the Case Closed box indicates that a case is closed.

Job 1

Change the Medisoft Program Date to June 23, 2010.

Print today's schedules for Dr. Crebore and Dr. Mahabir. Today is Wednesday, June 23, 2010.

Job 2

Susan Jonas accompanies Felidia, her daughter, for an appointment with Dr. Crebore. Felidia has been successfully treated for impetigo and needs a release to attend summer camp. Record the transactions using SD 50. Susan pays with check 2349. Print a walkout receipt.

Job 3

Cynthia Cashell is examined by Dr. Crebore for a flare-up of her psoriasis. Record the transaction using SD 51. Calculate the amount Cynthia owes, and enter her payment. She pays in full with check 102. Print a walkout receipt.

Job 4

Chantalle Usdan arrives for her sigmoidoscopy with Dr. Mahabir. Complete her patient information areas in Medisoft using SD 52. Create a new case. Since Chantalle is not a patient of Polaris Medical Group (she was referred by Dr. Rachel Innanni), a visit authorization number has been obtained by calling her insurance carrier. Enter authorization number 321404 in Medisoft.

Enter today's transactions using SD 53. Note that her diagnosis has been omitted from the encounter form—it is "other specified examination." Look up the ICD code, and enter the diagnosis in the Diagnosis tab of the Case folder. Enter Chantalle's copayment, which is made with check 409 (note that Dr. Mahabir is in the network). Print a walkout receipt.

❏ Internet Activity

Go to the website for CIGNA. Look up information on the different types of health plans offered. Explore the member and provider areas of the website.

❏ Job 5

A memo from the practice manager states that Jimmy LeConey's fever case and Roberta Yange-Sang's urinary tract infection case can now be closed. Close the cases.

❏ Job 6

Dr. Mahabir visits Rachel Atchely at Grandview Nursing Home. Rachel had cellulitis of the left foot and has been on a treatment regimen. Enter the transactions in Medisoft using SD 54. The copayment is paid with check 1078.

❏ Job 7

Mae Deysenrothe arrives at the office for a routine annual comprehensive physical examination with Dr. Mahabir. Create a new case. Record the transactions using SD 55. (*Optional:* Use the MultiLink feature to enter all the transactions except for the office visit code.) Payment is made with check 2043. Print a walkout receipt.

❏ Job 8

Hanna Wong calls to complain of chest pain when lifting. Hanna is not currently a patient of the practice but would like an appointment as soon as possible. Enter the following information, obtained over the phone, into the patient information section of Medisoft, and then schedule Hanna for a sixty-minute appointment at 10:00 tomorrow with Dr. Mahabir.

Hanna Z. Wong
22-B 22nd Avenue
Highland, OH 45132
Phone: 999-555-1122
Date of Birth: 11/5/37
Sex: F
SS#: 015-98-2139

❏ Job 9

Ann LeConey comes in for her appointment with Dr. Mahabir. He rechecks the irritated skin on her arm. Record the transactions using SD 56. The copayment is made with check 1834. Print a walkout receipt.

❏ Job 10

Print a patient day sheet for June 23, 2010.

❏ Job 11

Create insurance claims for June 23, 2010. Change the status of the claims.

Name _____ Date _____

Daily Worksheet

▰ WEEK 2
DAY 3

After completing all the jobs for Week 2 Day 3, answer the following questions in the spaces provided.

1. Who is the guarantor for Felidia Jonas's impetigo case?

   _____

   _____

2. Of the total charges for her June 23 office visit, for what amount is Cynthia Cashell responsible?

   _____

   _____

3. What is entered in the Visit Series Authorization Number box in the Account tab of the Case folder for Chantalle Usdan?

   _____

   _____

4. What is the charge for Rachel Atchely's nursing home visit on June 23?

   _____

   _____

5. What is the amount of Ann LeConey's copayment on June 23?

   _____

   _____

6. What is the total of all patient payments for June 23 (including copayments)?

   _____

   _____

7. How many insurance claims were created on June 23?

   _____

   _____

WEEK 2
DAY 4

Study the Medisoft Training Topic, and complete the jobs listed for today.

MEDISOFT TRAINING TOPIC 13:

Entering Additional Procedure Codes and Allowed Amounts

CPT codes are often updated and modified, and some are deleted. Before CPT codes can be selected in the Transaction Entry dialog box, they must be entered in the database. To add or modify CPT codes in Medisoft, select Procedure/Payment/Adjustment Codes from the Lists menu. The Procedure/Payment/Adjustment List dialog box is displayed. This box lists all the procedure, payment, and adjustment codes in the database. When the Field box at the top of the dialog box is set to Code 1 (the default), the codes are listed in numerical order. This setting can be changed to list the codes by description or type.

To add a new CPT code, click the New button at the bottom of the dialog box. The Procedure/Payment/Adjustment: (new) dialog box is displayed. The dialog box has three tabs: General, Amounts, and Allowed Amounts.

General Tab The General tab is used to enter detailed information about the code (see Figure T13-1). It contains the following fields:

FIGURE T13-1 General Tab of the Procedure/Payment/Adjustment Dialog Box

Code 1: The procedure code itself is entered in the Code 1 box. It can be from one to ten characters in length. After the code is entered and the Tab or Enter key is pressed, this code automatically appears in the Alternate Codes 2 and 3 boxes.

In some cases, these default entries in the Alternate Codes 2 and 3 boxes are deleted so that other alternate codes can be used. For example, some insurance carriers use different codes for the same procedure. The alternate code boxes allow these codes to be linked to the major code in Medisoft.

Inactive: Clicking the Inactive box designates a code as not in use. This option may be used when a code needs to be modified but open transactions (transactions that have not been returned to a zero balance) use the unmodified code. Codes marked as inactive appear with a red inactive message next to them in the Transaction Entry dialog box. Codes marked as inactive cannot be used unless the Inactive box is unchecked, making the code active again.

Description: In the Description box, enter an appropriate description of from one to forty characters.

Code Type: The Code Type drop-down list offers a number of choices for type of code, such as procedure charge, check copayment, adjustment, and insurance payment.

Account Code: Some practices group their procedure codes into account codes for reporting purposes. If an account code exists for the procedure code, it is entered in the Account Code box.

Type of Service: The appropriate type of service code is entered in the Type of Service box. Commonly used codes include:

1 Medical care

2 Surgery

3 Consultation

4 Diagnostic X-ray

5 Diagnostic lab

6 Radiation therapy

7 Anesthesia

8 Surgical assistance

9 Other medical

0 Blood charges

Place of Service: In the Place of Service box, enter the two-digit code that identifies the place the service was performed. Commonly used POS codes include:

11 Office

12 Home

21 Inpatient hospital

22 Outpatient hospital

23 Emergency room—hospital

24 Ambulatory surgical center

25 Birthing center

31 Skilled nursing facility

32 Nursing facility

33 Custodial care facility

Time To Do Procedure: Enter the approximate time, in minutes, required to perform the procedure. This information is used when determining the length of appointments scheduled in Office Hours. In the PMG database, only office visit procedure codes have been assigned time values.

Service Classification: This feature is available for assigning values (A-H) to procedures in order to classify them according to the category of service they represent. For example, A may be used for common procedures, B for surgery or lab charges, C for noncovered procedures, and so on. This feature is linked to the Insurance Coverage Percents by Service Classification field in the Policy tab of the Case dialog box, which determines the percentage of the charge amount that is billed to the insurance carrier as its share of the cost.

Don't Bill to Insurance: This feature allows you to restrict the printing of this particular code to certain insurance carriers. In the box, the code numbers of the insurance carriers that do not use this code are keyed. Enter the insurance carrier code numbers separated by commas.

Only Bill to Insurance: If a code is to be used only with certain insurance carriers, enter the codes of the insurance carriers, separated by commas.

Default Modifiers: If the procedure code always uses the same modifier(s), the modifiers can be entered in these boxes.

Revenue Code: If the practice is generating UB-04 claim forms, the revenue code for this procedure is entered.

Default Units: If applicable, the usual number of units for the procedure code can be entered.

The remaining fields are used in electronic claims:

National Drug Code: If the procedure has a national drug code assigned to it—for example, for reporting a prescription drug—the code is entered here.

Code ID Qualifier: If the National Drug Code has a qualifier indicating the type of code that is being transmitted, the qualifier is entered here.

Taxable: This box is clicked if the code requires a tax change.

HIPAA Approved: This box is linked to the Warn on Unapproved Codes option in the Program Options window. If the latter option is used, the HIPAA Approved box should be checked for each procedure code that is HIPAA compliant.

Require Co-pay: This box may be checked for a procedure that requires a copay (for example, an office visit code). When this box is checked for a code, whenever that code is entered in the Transaction Entry dialog box, the Co-pay box at the end of the transaction line displays a checkmark as a reminder that a copay is due.

Patient Only Responsible: A check in the Patient Only Responsible box indicates that no insurance claim forms will be generated. This box may be used when a patient's insurance policy is a capitated managed care plan.

Purchased Service: This box should be checked if the procedure is a service that is purchased from a third party—for example, lab work.

Amounts Tab   The Amounts tab contains information about the amount charged for the procedure (see Figure T13-2). It includes the following boxes:

Charge Amounts A to Z: The amount of the charge for the procedure is entered in the Charge Amounts A to Z boxes. Up to twenty-six different fees can be entered for each procedure. Box A is used to record the practice's normal charge for a procedure. Other boxes could be used to set up special pricing. For example, Box B could contain the fee for certain managed care plans that are paid a discounted amount, Box C could offer a standard discount for a cash payment, and so on.

FIGURE T13-2   Amounts Tab of the Procedure/Payment/Adjustment Dialog Box

The fees entered in the A to Z boxes are linked to the entry in the Price Code box in the Account tab within the Case folder. For example, if managed care fees are entered in the B box for each procedure code, managed care patients would also have B selected in the Price Code box. Then, when a charge is entered in the Transaction Entry dialog box, Medisoft automatically enters the fee listed in box B within the Amounts tab.

Polaris Medical Group uses a single fee schedule, so only box A is filled in. The actual amount the office receives for each procedure varies, however, depending on the type of insurance the patient has and the agreed-upon allowed amount for that procedure. The allowed amount paid by each carrier for a given procedure is entered in the Allowed Amounts tab of the Procedure/Payment/Adjustment dialog box, described below.

Cost of Service/Product: If there is an actual cost for the service or product, it is entered in the Cost of Service/Product box.

Medicare Allowed Amount: For Medicare participating providers, the allowed amount for this procedure can be entered in the Medicare Allowed Amount box. For nonparticipating providers, the Medicare limiting charge is entered. Medicare allowed amounts can also be entered in the Allowed Amounts tab for specific carriers.

Allowed Amounts The Allowed Amounts tab (see Figure T13-3) keeps track of the amount allowed for the procedure charge, sorted by insurance carrier. The allowed amount varies depending on the type of plan and the plan's arrangement with the practice. This tab can be completed and kept up to date by the practice, or it can be automatically calculated

FIGURE T13-3 Allowed Amounts Tab of the Procedure/Payment/Adjustment Dialog Box by Medisoft based on the latest payments received from the insurance company for a given procedure.

The amount each insurance carrier agrees to pay for the procedure is recorded in the Amount column to the right of the carrier's name.

When the information entered in the three tabs is complete, pressing the Save button saves the information in the database. The new code is now listed in the Procedure/Payment/Adjustment List dialog box and can be selected for use in the Transaction Entry dialog box.

❑ Job 1

Change the Medisoft Program Date to June 24, 2010.

Print today's schedules for Dr. Crebore and Dr. Mahabir. Today is Thursday, June 24, 2010.

❑ Job 2

Hanna Wong, a new Medicare patient, sees Dr. Mahabir for the chest pain she has been experiencing when lifting. Dr. Mahabir examines Hanna and would like her to return on June 30 for a series of tests of heart function.

Use SD 57 to enter Hanna's information in Medisoft and to create a new case. Then enter today's transactions using SD 58. Hanna pays the copayment with check 840. Print a walkout receipt. Finally, schedule Hanna for a sixty-minute appointment on June 30 at 2:00.

❑ Job 3

Will Brown telephones to inquire about the balance due on his account. Research the information, and inform him of the amount owed on his account, if any.

❑ Job 4

Review the audit/edit report found on SD 59. If there are any errors, correct them in Medisoft (for example, change an incorrect procedure code, an incorrect procedure charge, and so on).

❑ Job 5

Stewart Weintraub telephones. He is experiencing pain and stiffness in the arm that he fractured on June 16. Schedule him for a fifteen-minute appointment on June 29 at 3:15.

❏ Job 6

The practice manager has given you a list of new procedure codes (SD 60). Enter these codes in Medisoft. Fill in only those boxes for which information is provided on SD 60.

❏ Job 7

Jorge Martinez, a new patient, arrives for his appointment with Dr. Mahabir. He has been experiencing burning during urination. Using the information on SD 61, enter his information in Medisoft. Record the transactions, and enter the payment (made with check 1819) using SD 62. Print a walkout receipt.

❏ Job 8

Susan Jonas is examined by Dr. Crebore for a patch of contact dermatitis. When you try to enter the transaction from the encounter form (SD 63), you notice that no ICD code has been marked. Look in Susan's chart for today (SD 64) to locate the reason for her visit and a description of her diagnosis (Problem 1). Create a new case for the visit, and then locate the diagnosis code in Medisoft and enter it in the Diagnosis tab of the Case folder. Enter the transaction in Medisoft. Susan pays the copayment with check 349. Print a walkout receipt.

❏ Job 9

George Ahmadian telephones to request an appointment. He has a wart on his hand that he would like to have removed. Schedule him for a fifteen-minute appointment on June 28 at 9:45.

❏ Job 10

Print a patient day sheet for June 24, 2010.

❏ Job 11

Create insurance claims for June 24, 2010. Change the status of the claims.

Name _____ Date _____

Daily Worksheet

WEEK 2
DAY 4

After completing all the jobs for Week 2 Day 4, answer the following questions in the spaces provided.

1. What amount does Medicare owe for Hanna Wong's June 24 office visit after her copayment is deducted?

   _____

   _____

2. What is the amount William Brown owes on his account?

   _____

   _____

3. What is the description for procedure code 74290?

   _____

   _____

4. For what amount of Jorge Martinez's June 24 charges is his insurance carrier responsible after Martinez's copayment is deducted?

   _____

   _____

5. What is the amount of Susan Jonas's copayment on June 24?

   _____

   _____

6. What are the total procedure charges for June 24?

   _____

   _____

Study the Medisoft Training Topic, and complete the jobs listed for today.

MEDISOFT TRAINING TOPIC 14:

Using Final Draft, Medisoft's Integrated Word Processor

Medisoft contains a fully integrated word processing program called Final Draft. Final Draft can be used to enter patient notes and narratives as well as letters and other documents used by the practice. Data from the Medisoft program can also be pulled into a Final Draft document.

To use Final Draft, select the Final Draft option on the Activities menu. The main window of the program appears. To create a document, select New Document on the File menu (see Figure T14-1).

The menus on the menu bar at the top of the Final Draft window offer standard word processing features: text can be added, deleted, moved, copied, or replaced using the Edit menu; the default settings for font, line spacing, and page layout can be changed using the Format menu; and the spelling in a document can be checked using the Check Spelling option on the Tools menu. The File menu offers standard options for opening a new document,

FIGURE T14-1 Main Window of Final Draft Program with New Document Option Selected opening an existing document, saving a document (Save, Save As), and printing a document. It also contains an Import File option. Documents such as patient statements can be imported from the current practice that is open in Medisoft. To exit the program, select Exit on the File menu or click the X in the top right corner of the Final Draft window. When you exit, you are returned to the Medisoft program.

☑ Job 1

Change the Medisoft Program Date to June 25, 2010.

Print today's schedules for Dr. Crebore and Dr. Mahabir. Today is Friday, June 25, 2010.

☑ Job 2

Martin Szinovacz has his blood pressure checked by Dr. Crebore. Enter the transaction in Medisoft using SD 65.

☑ Job 3

Fran Ferrone calls for an appointment. She is still complaining of a cough that keeps her awake at night. Schedule her for a fifteen-minute appointment on June 30 at 3:45.

She also requests a copy of the office's Notice of Privacy Practices. Use the Final Draft word processor to write a short note that you will use as a cover letter when mailing the Notice of Privacy Practices brochure. Start the letter with Polaris Medical Group's address, followed by Fran Ferrone's address (see SD 39), and the date. The note should say, "Enclosed please find a copy of the Polaris Medical Group's Notice of Privacy Practices brochure, as requested. We look forward to seeing you at your next appointment on June 30." End the letter with your name and title (Patient Services Specialist). Print the letter, and then save it under the file name "Ferrone_cover." Select Letter as the File Type. When the Document Information dialog box appears, click OK to accept the default settings.

☑ Job 4

Eugene Kadar, a new patient, is examined by Dr. Crebore. Eugene is complaining of painful recurring sores on his lip. Using the information on SD 66, enter the information in Medisoft. Enter today's transactions using SD 67. Eugene pays with check 2039. Print a walkout receipt.

☑ Job 5

William Nisinson arrives at the office with workers' compensation paperwork. He is not a patient of PMG and does not have an appointment. He works for Dan's Hardware as a driver and has been injured on the job. While unloading a delivery, he fell off the back of the truck. A radiological examination by Dr. Mahabir reveals a fractured ankle, and a splint is applied.

Using SD 68, establish William as a patient in Medisoft. Additional information to be entered in the Case folder is as follows:

Policy tab: Dr. Mahabir accepts assignment. The insurance carrier pays 100 percent of charges (boxes A-H).

Condition tab: The date of the injury is June 25, 2010. It is employment-related. The accident is categorized as a Work injury/Non-collision. In the Dates Unable to Work section, enter *06/25/2010* in the From box.

Miscellaneous tab: Because this is a workers' compensation case, William must have an authorization number from his employer. Enter *Emp. Auth. #213-D* in the Local Use A box. (The remaining boxes in the Miscellaneous tab may be left blank.)

Then enter today's transactions using SD 69.

Also schedule William for a fifteen-minute follow-up appointment four weeks from today at 10:00.

☑ Internet Activity

Go to the website for the Ohio Bureau of Workers' Compensation. Look up information on the claim filing process.

☑ Job 6

Dan Connolly arrives for a follow-up visit for his hip pain with Dr. Mahabir. Enter the transactions using SD 70.

☑ Job 7

Yomo Hirosha, a patient of Dr. Mahabir, has been admitted to the Emergency Department of St. Mary's Hospital with complaints of chest pains. He has a history of myocardial infarction in April. Dr. Mahabir examines Yomo in the emergency room. Record the transaction in Medisoft using SD 71. Since this is a hospital visit, no copayment is collected.

❏ Job 8

Marilyn Rennagel arrives for her appointment with Dr. Crebore. Marilyn has changed jobs and insurance carriers since her last office visit. Using the information on SD 72, update her information in Medisoft. She has met her deductible with the new carrier. Then enter today's transactions using SD 73.

❏ Job 9

Will Brown arrives in the office without an appointment. He is experiencing rectal bleeding again and would like to see Dr. Mahabir. Dr. Mahabir is currently at St. Mary's Hospital, but Dr. Crebore can fit Will in after she is finished with her current patient. Record today's transactions from the encounter form (SD 74).

❏ Job 10

Wilma Estephan calls to report that she is still experiencing pain during urination. Schedule her for the first available fifteen-minute appointment with Dr. Mahabir on June 28.

❏ Job 11

An RA arrives with payment from Standard Health Care for Angelo Daiute's office visit on June 17, 2010 (SD 75). Compare the procedure codes and amounts with those in Medisoft. If they are correct, enter the payment in Medisoft.

❏ Job 12

Print a patient day sheet for June 25, 2010.

❏ Job 13

Create insurance claims for June 25, 2010. Change the status of the claims.

Name _____ Date _____

Daily Worksheet

WEEK 2
DAY 5

After completing all the jobs for Week 2 Day 5, answer the following questions in the spaces provided.

1. After her office visit on June 25, what amount does Marilyn Rennagel owe on her account?

   _____

   _____

2. What is the description for the ICD-9-CM code for Eugene Kadar's diagnosis?

   _____

   _____

3. What amount does Eugene Kadar's insurance carrier now owe for his June 25 office visit?

   _____

   _____

4. What is entered in the Local Use A box in the Miscellaneous tab of the Case folder for William Nisinson?

   _____

   _____

5. For what amount of Dan Connolly's June 25 charges is Medicare responsible?

   _____

   _____

6. What POS code is entered for Yomo Hirosha's transactions for June 25?

   _____

   _____

7. What code is entered in the Provider box in the Transaction Entry dialog box for William Brown's June 25 office visit?

   _____

   _____

8. What are the total insurance payments for June 25?

   _____

   _____

End-of-Month Jobs

Complete the jobs listed below.

❑ Job 1

Change the Medisoft Program Date to June 30, 2010, and use SDs 76 through 86 to enter the insurance payments in Medisoft.

Note: When applying payments in the Apply Payment/Adjustments to Charges screen, remember to tab across to the end of the each row so that the Remainder column (column 4) registers the payment fully.

❑ Job 2

Find all the patients who are insured under a CIGNA or Aetna capitated plan who were treated by Polaris Medical Group in May and June 2010. Since capitation payments arrived from CIGNA and Aetna, the charges in individual patient accounts must be written off so that patient accounts have zero balances.

Hint: In the Claim Management dialog box, the List Only button can be used to display only claims that match a specific insurance carrier. Use this button to display the list of patients insured under CIGNA and then Aetna who currently have claims. (Although capitated plans do not pay insurance claims, they request that claims be sent to them as they require the data for their records.) Make a note of each capitated patient's chart number for the two insurance carriers.

Then use the Enter Deposits/Payments option to enter a zero payment amount deposit for CIGNA. Select Insurance in the Payor Type field, select Electronic in the Payment Method field, and 0.00 in the Payment Amount field. Apply the zero amount deposit in the Apply Payment/Adjustments to Charges dialog box to adjust the account of each CIGNA patient to a zero balance by entering an amount in the *Adjustment* column equal to the amount already displayed in the *Remainder* column.

Create a zero payment amount deposit for Aetna, and follow the same steps to adjust the accounts for each Aetna patient.

After finishing your work in the Apply Payment/Adjustments to Charges dialog box for both groups of patients, change the status of the claims for these patients from Sent to Done.

Tip!

Job 2
Depending on the settings in the List Only Claims That Match dialog box (accessed through the List Only button), Done claims may or may not be listed along with other claims in the Claim Management dialog box. To include Done claims in the display, click the List Only button in the Claim Management dialog box to display the List Only Claims That Match dialog box. In the Claim Status section, make sure the Exclude Done checkbox is not checked.

❑ Job 3

Create remainder statements for all patients with outstanding balances greater than $5.00. Change the status of the statements from Ready to Send to Sent.

❏ Job 4

Using the patient day sheets for June 14 through 25, add up the total charges, receipts, and adjustments for the ten-day period. Make a note of these totals.

Now print a practice analysis report for June 14 through 25, 2010. Add the total charges, payments, and adjustments.

Compare the totals on the practice analysis with the totals for the day sheets you have for the same time period. The amounts on the practice analysis should agree with the amounts from the totaled day sheets.

❏ Job 5

Print a patient aging report through June 30, 2010. *Note:* Be sure to use the Patient Aging Applied Payment report rather than the Patient Aging report for this job.

Part 4

Source Documents

This section contains the source documents referred to in Part 3, On the Job. These documents represent typical paperwork found in medical practices, and include patient information forms, encounter forms, physician's notes, chart notes, remittance advices, and audit/edit reports. Following is a numerical list of the source documents in Part 4:

Doc. No.	Page No.	Form Type	Subject
1	168	Patient Information	Mary Anne Kopelman
2	169	Encounter	Mary Anne Kopelman
3	170	RA	Medicare
4	171	Encounter	Lydia Stephanos
5	172	Patient Information	Gregory Kavanaugh
6	173	Encounter	Gregory Kavanaugh
7	174	RA	Standard Health Care
8	175	Encounter	Daniel Connolly
9	176	Patient Information	Wilma Estephan
10	177	Encounter	Wilma Estephan
11	178	Patient Information	James LeConey
12	179	Encounter	James LeConey
13	180	Encounter	William Brown
14	181	RA	Ohio Insurance Company
15	182	Encounter	Alan Harcar
16	183	Patient Information	Nora McAniff
17	184	Encounter	Nora McAniff
18	185	RA	Blue Cross Blue Shield
19	186	Physician's Notes	Stewart Weintraub
20	187	RA	Medicare
21	188	Encounter	George Ahmadian
22	189	Encounter	Victoria Ferrara
23	190	New Provider Notes	Dr. Sylvia T. Serto
24	191	RA	Standard Health Care
25	192	Patient Information	Angelo Daiute
26	193	Encounter	Angelo Daiute
27	194	Encounter	Cameron Trotta

28	195	Encounter	George Ahmadian
29	196	RA	Standard Health Care
30	197	Patient Information	Hector Valaquez
31	198	Encounter	Hector Valaquez
32	199	Encounter	Seymour Colbs
33	200	Encounter	David Weatherly
34	201	Audit/Edit Report	Medicare
35	202	Encounter	Roberta Yange-Sang
36	203	Encounter	Gloria Berkel-Rees
37	204	Encounter	Alan Harcar
38	205	Physician's Notes	Myrna Beedon
39	206	Patient Information	Fran Ferrone
40	207	Encounter	Fran Ferrone
41	208	Encounter	Jimmy Hellery
42	209	Encounter	Floyd Deysenrothe
43	210	RA	Blue Cross Blue Shield
44	211	Encounter	Elizabeth Wu
45	212	ICD Codes	Additions
46	213	Encounter	Flora Torres-Gil
47	214	New Carrier Notes	Ohio Maxcare PPO
48	215	New Carrier Fee Schedule	Ohio Maxcare PPO
49	216	Encounter	Diana O'Keefe
50	217	Encounter	Felidia Jonas
51	218	Encounter	Cynthia Cashell
52	219	Patient Information	Chantalle Usdan
53	220	Encounter	Chantalle Usdan
54	221	Encounter	Rachel Atchely
55	222	Encounter	Mae Deysenrothe
56	223	Encounter	Ann LeConey
57	224	Patient Information	Hanna Wong
58	225	Encounter	Hanna Wong
59	226	Audit/Edit Report	Medicare
60	227	CPT Codes	Additions
61	228	Patient Information	Jorge Martinez
62	229	Encounter	Jorge Martinez
63	230	Encounter	Susan Jonas
64	231	Chart Notes	Susan Jonas
65	232	Encounter	Martin Szinovacz
66	233	Patient Information	Eugene Kadar
67	234	Encounter	Eugene Kadar
68	235	Patient Information	William Nisinson
69	236	Encounter	William Nisinson
70	237	Encounter	Daniel Connolly

71	238	Physician's Notes	Yomo Hirosha
72	239	Patient Information	Marilyn Rennagel
73	240	Encounter	Marilyn Rennagel
74	241	Encounter	William Brown
75	242	RA	Standard Health Care
76	243	RA	Ohio Insurance Company
77	244	RA	Standard Health Care
78	245	RA	Blue Cross Blue Shield
79	246	RA	Workers' Compensation
80	247	RA	Medicare HMO
81	248	RA	TRICARE
82	249	RA	Medicare
83	250	RA	Medicaid
84	251	RA	Columbus Medical Care
85	252	RA	Aetna
86	253	RA	CIGNA

PATIENT INFORMATION FORM

THIS SECTION REFERS TO PATIENT ONLY

Name: Mary Anne C. Kopelman	Sex: F	Marital Status: ☐S ☒M ☐D ☐W	Birth Date: 9/7/79

Address: 45 Mason Street	SS#: 465-99-0022	

City: Hopewell	State: OH	Zip: 43746	Employer:	Phone:

Home Phone: 999-555-6877	Employer's Address:

Work Phone:	City:	State:	Zip:

Spouse's Name: Arnold B. Kopelman	Spouse's Employer: U.S. Army, Fort Tyrone

Emergency Contact: Arnold B. Kopelman	Relationship: Husband	Phone #: 999-555-0018

FILL IN IF PATIENT IS A MINOR

Parent/Guardian's Name:	Sex:	Marital Status: ☐S ☐M ☐D ☐W	Birth Date:

Phone:	SS#:	

Address:	Employer:	Phone:

City:	State:	Zip:	Employer's Address:

Student Status:	City:	State:	Zip:

INSURANCE INFORMATION

Primary Insurance Company: TRICARE	Secondary Insurance Company:

Subscriber's Name: Arnold B. Kopelman	Birth Date: 4/10/79	Subscriber's Name:	Birth Date:

Plan: TRICARE	SS#: 230-56-9874	Plan:

Policy #: 230-56-9874	Group #: USA9947	Policy #:	Group #:

Copayment/Deductible: $10 copay	Price Code: A	

OTHER INFORMATION

Reason for visit: shortness of breath, fatigue	Allergy to Medication (list):

Name of referring physician:	If auto accident, list date and state in which it occurred:

I authorize treatment and agree to pay all fees and charges for the person named above. I agree to pay all charges shown by statements, promptly upon their presentation, unless credit arrangements are agreed upon in writing.

I authorize payment directly to POLARIS MEDICAL GROUP of insurance benefits otherwise payable to me. I hereby authorize the release of any medical information necessary in order to process a claim for payment in my behalf.

Mary Anne Kopelman	6/14/10
(Patient's Signature/Parent or Guardian's Signature)	(Date)

I plan to make payment of my medical expenses as follows (check one or more):

__X__ Insurance (as above)   __X__ Cash/Check/Credit/Debit Card   _____ Medicare   _____ Medicaid   _____ Workers' Comp.

ENCOUNTER FORM

6/14/2010 DATE	**10:00am** TIME
Mary Anne C. Kopelman PATIENT NAME	

Dr. Robin Crebore
PROVIDER

KOPELMA0
CHART #

OFFICE VISITS - SYMPTOMATIC - NEW		
99201	OF--New Patient Minimal	
99202	OF--New Patient Low	X
99203	OF--New Patient Detailed	
99204	OF--New Patient Moderate	
99205	OF--New Patient High	

OFFICE VISITS - SYMPTOMATIC - ESTABLISHED		
99211	OF--Established Patient Minimal	
99212	OF--Established Patient Low	
99213	OF--Established Patient Detailed	
99214	OF--Established Patient Moderate	
99215	OF--Established Patient High	

PREVENTIVE VISITS - NEW		
99381	Under 1 Year	
99382	1 - 4 Years	
99383	5 - 11 Years	
99384	12 - 17 Years	
99385	18 - 39 Years	
99386	40 - 64 Years	
99387	65 Years & Up	

PREVENTIVE VISITS - ESTABLISHED		
99391	Under 1 Year	
99392	1 - 4 Years	
99393	5 - 11 Years	
99394	12 - 17 Years	
99395	18 - 39 Years	
99396	40 - 64 Years	
99397	65 Years & Up	

HOSPITAL/NURSING HOME VISITS		
99221	Initial hospital care, det.	
99222	Initial hospital care, comp.	
99223	Initial hospital care, high	
99281	ER Visit, min.	
99282	ER Visit, low	
99283	ER Visit, det.	
99284	ER Visit, moderate	
99285	ER Visit, high	
99307	Subseq. nursing facility care, pf.	

PROCEDURES		
10060	Incision/drainage, abcess	
20610	Aspiration, bursa	
29505	Splint, long leg	
29515	Splint, short leg	
36415	Routine venipuncture	X
45330	Sigmoidoscopy, flex	
46600	Anoscopy, diagnostic	
71030	Chest x-ray, complete	
73610	Radiology, ankle, complete	
93000	Routine ECG	
93018	Cardiovascular stress test	
99070	Supplies and materials	

LABORATORY		
80050	General health panel	X
81000	Urinalysis, complete	
82270	Blood, occult, feces screening	
82607	Vitamin B-12 test	
82948	Glucose, blood reagent	
85027	CBC, automated	
85651	Sedimentation rate test, manual	
86360	Absolute CD4/CD8 ratio	
86592	Syphilis test	
87070	Throat culture	
87088	Urine culture	
88150	Cytopathology, cervical or vaginal	

INJECTIONS		
90471	Immunization administration	
90472	Immunization administration, 2nd	
90658	Influenza injection, ages >3	
90702	DT immunization, ages <7	
90703	Tetanus immunization	
90707	MMR immunization	
90722	Therapeutic injection	
90723	DtaP - HepB - IPV	
90732	Pneumococcal immunization	

POLARIS MEDICAL GROUP

REFERRING PHYSICIAN	NPI	NOTES
AUTHORIZATION #		
DIAGNOSIS 280.9		
PAYMENT AMOUNT $10 copay, check #1011		

Nationwide Medicare
P.O. Box 7000
Columbus, OH 43214

Polaris Medical Group
2100 Grace Avenue
Columbus, OH 43214

Practice ID: 10-123456

Date Prepared : 6/10/10   **EFT Number:** 3642987

Patient's Name	Dates of Service From - Thru	POS	Proc	Qty	Charge Amount	Allowed Amount	Patient Resp.	Amt. Paid Provider
Stephanos, Lydia	05/27/10 - 05/27/10	11	99397	1	$155.00	$118.00	$118.00	$00.00**
Stephanos, Lydia	05/27/10 - 05/27/10	11	93000	1	$84.00	$29.00	$5.80	$23.20

**96: This procedure is not covered by Nationwide Medicare.

* * * * * * *   *EFT transmitted in the amount of $23.20*   * * * * * * *

ENCOUNTER FORM

6/14/2010	10:00am		Dr. Michael Mahabir
DATE	TIME		PROVIDER
Lydia Stephanos			STEPHLY0
PATIENT NAME			CHART #

OFFICE VISITS - SYMPTOMATIC - NEW		
99201	OF--New Patient Minimal	
99202	OF--New Patient Low	
99203	OF--New Patient Detailed	
99204	OF--New Patient Moderate	
99205	OF--New Patient High	

OFFICE VISITS - SYMPTOMATIC - ESTABLISHED		
99211	OF--Established Patient Minimal	
99212	OF--Established Patient Low	
99213	OF--Established Patient Detailed	X
99214	OF--Established Patient Moderate	
99215	OF--Established Patient High	

PREVENTIVE VISITS - NEW		
99381	Under 1 Year	
99382	1 - 4 Years	
99383	5 - 11 Years	
99384	12 - 17 Years	
99385	18 - 39 Years	
99386	40 - 64 Years	
99387	65 Years & Up	

PREVENTIVE VISITS - ESTABLISHED		
99391	Under 1 Year	
99392	1 - 4 Years	
99393	5 - 11 Years	
99394	12 - 17 Years	
99395	18 - 39 Years	
99396	40 - 64 Years	
99397	65 Years & Up	

HOSPITAL/NURSING HOME VISITS		
99221	Initial hospital care, det.	
99222	Initial hospital care, comp.	
99223	Initial hospital care, high	
99281	ER Visit, min.	
99282	ER Visit, low	
99283	ER Visit, det.	
99284	ER Visit, moderate	
99285	ER Visit, high	
99307	Subseq. nursing facility care, pf.	

PROCEDURES		
10060	Incision/drainage, abcess	X
20610	Aspiration, bursa	
29505	Splint, long leg	
29515	Splint, short leg	
36415	Routine venipuncture	
45330	Sigmoidoscopy, flex	
46600	Anoscopy, diagnostic	
71030	Chest x-ray, complete	
73610	Radiology, ankle, complete	
93000	Routine ECG	
93018	Cardiovascular stress test	
99070	Supplies and materials	

LABORATORY		
80050	General health panel	
81000	Urinalysis, complete	
82270	Blood, occult, feces screening	
82607	Vitamin B-12 test	
82948	Glucose, blood reagent	
85027	CBC, automated	
85651	Sedimentation rate test, manual	
86360	Absolute CD4/CD8 ratio	
86592	Syphilis test	
87070	Throat culture	
87088	Urine culture	
88150	Cytopathology, cervical or vaginal	

INJECTIONS		
90471	Immunization administration	
90472	Immunization administration, 2nd	
90658	Influenza injection, ages >3	
90702	DT immunization, ages <7	
90703	Tetanus immunization	
90707	MMR immunization	
90722	Therapeutic injection	
90723	DtaP - HepB - IPV	
90732	Pneumococcal immunization	

POLARIS MEDICAL GROUP

REFERRING PHYSICIAN		NPI		NOTES
AUTHORIZATION #				
DIAGNOSIS				
706.2				
PAYMENT AMOUNT				

PATIENT INFORMATION FORM

THIS SECTION REFERS TO PATIENT ONLY

Name: Gregory Kavanaugh	Sex: M	Marital Status: ☒S ☐M ☐D ☐W	Birth Date: 12/15/84

Address: 54 Grove St., Apt. 20			SS#: 677-98-0078	

City: Germantown	State: OH	Zip: 45327	Employer: Computer Consultants	Phone: 999-555-3333

Home Phone: 999-555-2626	Employer's Address: 130 Parkway South

Work Phone:	City: Columbus	State: OH	Zip: 43214

Spouse's Name:	Spouse's Employer:

Emergency Contact: Ron Kavanaugh	Relationship: brother	Phone #: 999-555-0036

FILL IN IF PATIENT IS A MINOR

Parent/Guardian's Name:	Sex:	Marital Status: ☐S ☐M ☐D ☐W	Birth Date:

Phone:	SS#:

Address:	Employer:	Phone:

City:	State:	Zip:	Employer's Address:

Student Status:	City:	State:	Zip:

INSURANCE INFORMATION

Primary Insurance Company: Standard Health Care, Inc.	Secondary Insurance Company:

Subscriber's Name: Gregory Kavanaugh	Birth Date: 12/15/84	Subscriber's Name:	Birth Date:

Plan: PPO	SS#: 677-98-0078	Plan:

Policy #: 000-GK9878	Group #: CCTAA	Policy #:	Group #:

Copayment/Deductible: $15 / $1,000	Price Code: A	

OTHER INFORMATION

Reason for visit: routine monitoring	Allergy to Medication (list):

Name of referring physician:	If auto accident, list date and state in which it occurred:

I authorize treatment and agree to pay all fees and charges for the person named above. I agree to pay all charges shown by statements, promptly upon their presentation, unless credit arrangements are agreed upon in writing.

I authorize payment directly to POLARIS MEDICAL GROUP of insurance benefits otherwise payable to me. I hereby authorize the release of any medical information necessary in order to process a claim for payment in my behalf.

Gregory Kavanaugh	6/14/10
(Patient's Signature/Parent or Guardian's Signature)	(Date)

I plan to make payment of my medical expenses as follows (check one or more):

__X__ Insurance (as above)   __X__ Cash/Check/Credit/Debit Card   _____ Medicare   _____ Medicaid   _____ Workers' Comp.

ENCOUNTER FORM

6/14/2010 **10:30am**	**Dr. Robin Crebore**
DATE TIME	PROVIDER
Gregory Kavanaugh	**KAVANGR0**
PATIENT NAME	CHART #

OFFICE VISITS - SYMPTOMATIC - NEW		
99201	OF--New Patient Minimal	
99202	OF--New Patient Low	
99203	OF--New Patient Detailed	
99204	OF--New Patient Moderate	
99205	OF--New Patient High	
OFFICE VISITS - SYMPTOMATIC - ESTABLISHED		
99211	OF--Established Patient Minimal	
99212	OF--Established Patient Low	X
99213	OF--Established Patient Detailed	
99214	OF--Established Patient Moderate	
99215	OF--Established Patient High	
PREVENTIVE VISITS - NEW		
99381	Under 1 Year	
99382	1 - 4 Years	
99383	5 - 11 Years	
99384	12 - 17 Years	
99385	18 - 39 Years	
99386	40 - 64 Years	
99387	65 Years & Up	
PREVENTIVE VISITS - ESTABLISHED		
99391	Under 1 Year	
99392	1 - 4 Years	
99393	5 - 11 Years	
99394	12 - 17 Years	
99395	18 - 39 Years	
99396	40 - 64 Years	
99397	65 Years & Up	
HOSPITAL/NURSING HOME VISITS		
99221	Initial hospital care, det.	
99222	Initial hospital care, comp.	
99223	Initial hospital care, high	
99281	ER Visit, min.	
99282	ER Visit, low	
99283	ER Visit, det.	
99284	ER Visit, moderate	
99285	ER Visit, high	
99307	Subseq. nursing facility care, pf.	

PROCEDURES		
10060	Incision/drainage, abcess	
20610	Aspiration, bursa	
29505	Splint, long leg	
29515	Splint, short leg	
36415	Routine venipuncture	X
45330	Sigmoidoscopy, flex	
46600	Anoscopy, diagnostic	
71030	Chest x-ray, complete	
73610	Radiology, ankle, complete	
93000	Routine ECG	
93018	Cardiovascular stress test	
99070	Supplies and materials	
LABORATORY		
80050	General health panel	
81000	Urinalysis, complete	
82270	Blood, occult, feces screening	
82607	Vitamin B-12 test	
82948	Glucose, blood reagent	
85027	CBC, automated	
85651	Sedimentation rate test, manual	
86360	Absolute CD4/CD8 ratio	X
86592	Syphilis test	
87070	Throat culture	
87088	Urine culture	
88150	Cytopathology, cervical or vaginal	
INJECTIONS		
90471	Immunization administration	
90472	Immunization administration, 2nd	
90658	Influenza injection, ages >3	
90702	DT immunization, ages <7	
90703	Tetanus immunization	
90707	MMR immunization	
90722	Therapeutic injection	
90723	DtaP - HepB - IPV	
90732	Pneumococcal immunization	

POLARIS MEDICAL GROUP		NOTES
REFERRING PHYSICIAN	NPI	
AUTHORIZATION #		
DIAGNOSIS 042		
PAYMENT AMOUNT $15 copay, check #200		

Standard Health Care
1500 Summit Avenue, Suite 500
Cincinnati, OH 45000

Polaris Medical Group
2100 Grace Avenue
Columbus, OH 43214

Practice ID: 01-234567

Date Prepared: 6/14/10   EFT Number: 267498

Patient's Name	Dates of Service From - Thru	POS	Proc	Qty	Charge Amount	Allowed Amount	Patient Resp.	Amt. Paid Provider
Szinovacz, Martin	5/19/10 - 5/19/10	11	99213	1	$72.00	$62.00	$15.00	$47.00

* * * * * * * *   *EFT transmitted in the amount of $47.00*   * * * * * * * *

ENCOUNTER FORM

6/14/2010　　　**2:00pm**	**Dr. Michael Mahabir**
DATE　　　　　　TIME	PROVIDER
Daniel Connolly	**CONNODA0**
PATIENT NAME	CHART #

OFFICE VISITS - SYMPTOMATIC - NEW		
99201	OF--New Patient Minimal	
99202	OF--New Patient Low	
99203	OF--New Patient Detailed	
99204	OF--New Patient Moderate	
99205	OF--New Patient High	

OFFICE VISITS - SYMPTOMATIC - ESTABLISHED		
99211	OF--Established Patient Minimal	
99212	OF--Established Patient Low	
99213	OF--Established Patient Detailed	
99214	OF--Established Patient Moderate	X
99215	OF--Established Patient High	

PREVENTIVE VISITS - NEW		
99381	Under 1 Year	
99382	1 - 4 Years	
99383	5 - 11 Years	
99384	12 - 17 Years	
99385	18 - 39 Years	
99386	40 - 64 Years	
99387	65 Years & Up	

PREVENTIVE VISITS - ESTABLISHED		
99391	Under 1 Year	
99392	1 - 4 Years	
99393	5 - 11 Years	
99394	12 - 17 Years	
99395	18 - 39 Years	
99396	40 - 64 Years	
99397	65 Years & Up	

HOSPITAL/NURSING HOME VISITS		
99221	Initial hospital care, det.	
99222	Initial hospital care, comp.	
99223	Initial hospital care, high	
99281	ER Visit, min.	
99282	ER Visit, low	
99283	ER Visit, det.	
99284	ER Visit, moderate	
99285	ER Visit, high	
99307	Subseq. nursing facility care, pf.	

PROCEDURES		
10060	Incision/drainage, abcess	
20610	Aspiration, bursa	
29505	Splint, long leg	
29515	Splint, short leg	
36415	Routine venipuncture	
45330	Sigmoidoscopy, flex	
46600	Anoscopy, diagnostic	
71030	Chest x-ray, complete	
73610	Radiology, ankle, complete	
93000	Routine ECG	
93018	Cardiovascular stress test	
99070	Supplies and materials	

LABORATORY		
80050	General health panel	
81000	Urinalysis, complete	
82270	Blood, occult, feces screening	
82607	Vitamin B-12 test	
82948	Glucose, blood reagent	
85027	CBC, automated	
85651	Sedimentation rate test, manual	
86360	Absolute CD4/CD8 ratio	
86592	Syphilis test	
87070	Throat culture	
87088	Urine culture	
88150	Cytopathology, cervical or vaginal	

INJECTIONS		
90471	Immunization administration	
90472	Immunization administration, 2nd	
90658	Influenza injection, ages >3	
90702	DT immunization, ages <7	
90703	Tetanus immunization	
90707	MMR immunization	
90722	Therapeutic injection	
90723	DtaP - HepB - IPV	
90732	Pneumococcal immunization	

POLARIS MEDICAL GROUP		NOTES
REFERRING PHYSICIAN	NPI	
AUTHORIZATION #		
DIAGNOSIS 719.45		
PAYMENT AMOUNT		

PATIENT INFORMATION FORM

THIS SECTION REFERS TO PATIENT ONLY

Name: Wilma Estephan	Sex: F	Marital Status: ☐ S ☐ M ☐ D ☒ W	Birth Date: 1/9/25

Address: 22 Horace Mann Road	SS#: 009-10-9988

City: Highland	State: OH	Zip: 45132	Employer:	Phone:

Home Phone: 999-555-2387	Employer's Address:

Work Phone:	City:	State:	Zip:

Spouse's Name:	Spouse's Employer:

Emergency Contact: Joan Hause	Relationship: daughter	Phone #: 999-302-4609

FILL IN IF PATIENT IS A MINOR

Parent/Guardian's Name:	Sex:	Marital Status: ☐ S ☐ M ☐ D ☐ W	Birth Date:

Phone:	SS#:

Address:	Employer:	Phone:

City:	State:	Zip:	Employer's Address:

Student Status:	City:	State:	Zip:

INSURANCE INFORMATION

Primary Insurance Company: Nationwide Medicare	Secondary Insurance Company:

Subscriber's Name: Wilma Estephan	Birth Date: 1-9-25	Subscriber's Name:	Birth Date:

Plan: HMO	SS#: 009-10-9988	Plan:

Policy #: 009-10-9988A	Group #:	Policy #:	Group #:

Copayment/Deductible: $5 copay	Price Code: A	

OTHER INFORMATION

Reason for visit: pain upon urination	Allergy to Medication (list):

Name of referring physician:	If auto accident, list date and state in which it occurred:

I authorize treatment and agree to pay all fees and charges for the person named above. I agree to pay all charges shown by statements, promptly upon their presentation, unless credit arrangements are agreed upon in writing.

I authorize payment directly to POLARIS MEDICAL GROUP of insurance benefits otherwise payable to me. I hereby authorize the release of any medical information necessary in order to process a claim for payment in my behalf.

Wilma Estephan	6/15/10
(Patient's Signature/Parent or Guardian's Signature)	(Date)

I plan to make payment of my medical expenses as follows (check one or more):

_____ Insurance (as above)   __X__ Cash/Check/Credit/Debit Card   __X__ Medicare   _____ Medicaid   _____ Workers' Comp.

ENCOUNTER FORM

6/15/2010 **9:30am**	**Dr. Michael Mahabir**
DATE TIME	PROVIDER
Wilma T. Estephan	**ESTEPWI0**
PATIENT NAME	CHART #

OFFICE VISITS - SYMPTOMATIC - NEW		
99201	OF--New Patient Minimal	
99202	OF--New Patient Low	X
99203	OF--New Patient Detailed	
99204	OF--New Patient Moderate	
99205	OF--New Patient High	

OFFICE VISITS - SYMPTOMATIC - ESTABLISHED		
99211	OF--Established Patient Minimal	
99212	OF--Established Patient Low	
99213	OF--Established Patient Detailed	
99214	OF--Established Patient Moderate	
99215	OF--Established Patient High	

PREVENTIVE VISITS - NEW		
99381	Under 1 Year	
99382	1 - 4 Years	
99383	5 - 11 Years	
99384	12 - 17 Years	
99385	18 - 39 Years	
99386	40 - 64 Years	
99387	65 Years & Up	

PREVENTIVE VISITS - ESTABLISHED		
99391	Under 1 Year	
99392	1 - 4 Years	
99393	5 - 11 Years	
99394	12 - 17 Years	
99395	18 - 39 Years	
99396	40 - 64 Years	
99397	65 Years & Up	

HOSPITAL/NURSING HOME VISITS		
99221	Initial hospital care, det.	
99222	Initial hospital care, comp.	
99223	Initial hospital care, high	
99281	ER Visit, min.	
99282	ER Visit, low	
99283	ER Visit, det.	
99284	ER Visit, moderate	
99285	ER Visit, high	
99307	Subseq. nursing facility care, pf.	

PROCEDURES		
10060	Incision/drainage, abcess	
20610	Aspiration, bursa	
29505	Splint, long leg	
29515	Splint, short leg	
36415	Routine venipuncture	
45330	Sigmoidoscopy, flex	
46600	Anoscopy, diagnostic	
71030	Chest x-ray, complete	
73610	Radiology, ankle, complete	
93000	Routine ECG	
93018	Cardiovascular stress test	
99070	Supplies and materials	

LABORATORY		
80050	General health panel	
81000	Urinalysis, complete	X
82270	Blood, occult, feces screening	
82607	Vitamin B-12 test	
82948	Glucose, blood reagent	
85027	CBC, automated	
85651	Sedimentation rate test, manual	
86360	Absolute CD4/CD8 ratio	
86592	Syphilis test	
87070	Throat culture	
87088	Urine culture	X
88150	Cytopathology, cervical or vaginal	

INJECTIONS		
90471	Immunization administration	
90472	Immunization administration, 2nd	
90658	Influenza injection, ages >3	
90702	DT immunization, ages <7	
90703	Tetanus immunization	
90707	MMR immunization	
90722	Therapeutic injection	
90723	DtaP - HepB - IPV	
90732	Pneumococcal immunization	

POLARIS MEDICAL GROUP

		NOTES
REFERRING PHYSICIAN	NPI	
AUTHORIZATION #		
DIAGNOSIS
595.2		
PAYMENT AMOUNT
$5 copay, check #359		

PATIENT INFORMATION FORM

THIS SECTION REFERS TO PATIENT ONLY

Name: Jimmy LeConey	Sex: M	Marital Status: ☒S ☐M ☐D ☐W	Birth Date: 6/30/94

Address: 27 Ballard Drive	SS#: 887-68-4256	

City: Fairview	State: OH	Zip: 43773	Employer:	Phone:

Home Phone: 999-555-2398	Employer's Address:

Work Phone:	City:	State:	Zip:

Spouse's Name:	Spouse's Employer:

Emergency Contact: Ann LeConey	Relationship: mother	Phone #: 999-555-2398

FILL IN IF PATIENT IS A MINOR

Parent/Guardian's Name: Brian Howard (father)	Sex: M	Marital Status: ☐S ☐M ☒D ☐W	Birth Date: 1/8/65

Phone: 999-555-3124	SS#: 350-26-0419	

Address: 2349 Sheffield Way	Employer: Columbus World Press, full-time	Phone:

City: Columbus	State: OH	Zip: 43214	Employer's Address: 2399 Overland Way

Student Status:	City: Columbus	State: OH	Zip: 43214

INSURANCE INFORMATION

Primary Insurance Company: Blue Cross & Blue Shield of Ohio	Secondary Insurance Company:

Subscriber's Name: Brian Howard	Birth Date: 1/8/65	Subscriber's Name:	Birth Date:

Plan: Traditional	SS#: 350-26-0419	Plan:

Policy #: XGS7612979	Group #: 67544	Policy #:	Group #:

Copayment/Deductible: $500 deductible	Price Code: A	

OTHER INFORMATION

Reason for visit: flu	Allergy to Medication (list):

Name of referring physician:	If auto accident, list date and state in which it occurred:

I authorize treatment and agree to pay all fees and charges for the person named above. I agree to pay all charges shown by statements, promptly upon their presentation, unless credit arrangements are agreed upon in writing.

I authorize payment directly to POLARIS MEDICAL GROUP of insurance benefits otherwise payable to me. I hereby authorize the release of any medical information necessary in order to process a claim for payment in my behalf.

Ann LeConey	6/15/10
(Patient's Signature/Parent or Guardian's Signature)	(Date)

I plan to make payment of my medical expenses as follows (check one or more):

__X__ Insurance (as above)   __X__ Cash/Check/Credit/Debit Card   _____ Medicare   _____ Medicaid   _____ Workers' Comp.

ENCOUNTER FORM

6/15/2010	9:30am		Dr. Michael Mahabir
DATE	TIME		PROVIDER

James I. LeConey		LECONJI0
PATIENT NAME		CHART #

OFFICE VISITS - SYMPTOMATIC - NEW		
99201	OF--New Patient Minimal	
99202	OF--New Patient Low	
99203	OF--New Patient Detailed	
99204	OF--New Patient Moderate	
99205	OF--New Patient High	
OFFICE VISITS - SYMPTOMATIC - ESTABLISHED		
99211	OF--Established Patient Minimal	
99212	OF--Established Patient Low	
99213	OF--Established Patient Detailed	
99214	OF--Established Patient Moderate	X
99215	OF--Established Patient High	
PREVENTIVE VISITS - NEW		
99381	Under 1 Year	
99382	1 - 4 Years	
99383	5 - 11 Years	
99384	12 - 17 Years	
99385	18 - 39 Years	
99386	40 - 64 Years	
99387	65 Years & Up	
PREVENTIVE VISITS - ESTABLISHED		
99391	Under 1 Year	
99392	1 - 4 Years	
99393	5 - 11 Years	
99394	12 - 17 Years	
99395	18 - 39 Years	
99396	40 - 64 Years	
99397	65 Years & Up	
HOSPITAL/NURSING HOME VISITS		
99221	Initial hospital care, det.	
99222	Initial hospital care, comp.	
99223	Initial hospital care, high	
99281	ER Visit, min.	
99282	ER Visit, low	
99283	ER Visit, det.	
99284	ER Visit, moderate	
99285	ER Visit, high	
99307	Subseq. nursing facility care, pf.	

PROCEDURES		
10060	Incision/drainage, abcess	
20610	Aspiration, bursa	
29505	Splint, long leg	
29515	Splint, short leg	
36415	Routine venipuncture	
45330	Sigmoidoscopy, flex	
46600	Anoscopy, diagnostic	
71030	Chest x-ray, complete	
73610	Radiology, ankle, complete	
93000	Routine ECG	
93018	Cardiovascular stress test	
99070	Supplies and materials	
LABORATORY		
80050	General health panel	
81000	Urinalysis, complete	
82270	Blood, occult, feces screening	
82607	Vitamin B-12 test	
82948	Glucose, blood reagent	
85027	CBC, automated	
85651	Sedimentation rate test, manual	
86360	Absolute CD4/CD8 ratio	
86592	Syphilis test	
87070	Throat culture	
87088	Urine culture	
88150	Cytopathology, cervical or vaginal	
INJECTIONS		
90471	Immunization administration	
90472	Immunization administration, 2nd	
90658	Influenza injection, ages >3	
90702	DT immunization, ages <7	
90703	Tetanus immunization	
90707	MMR immunization	
90722	Therapeutic injection	
90723	DtaP - HepB - IPV	
90732	Pneumococcal immunization	

POLARIS MEDICAL GROUP

REFERRING PHYSICIAN	NPI	NOTES
AUTHORIZATION #		
DIAGNOSIS **487.1**		
PAYMENT AMOUNT		

ENCOUNTER FORM

6/15/2010	9:30am	Dr. Michael Mahabir
DATE	TIME	PROVIDER
William A. Brown		BROWNWI0
PATIENT NAME		CHART #

OFFICE VISITS - SYMPTOMATIC - NEW		
99201	OF--New Patient Minimal	
99202	OF--New Patient Low	
99203	OF--New Patient Detailed	
99204	OF--New Patient Moderate	
99205	OF--New Patient High	
OFFICE VISITS - SYMPTOMATIC - ESTABLISHED		
99211	OF--Established Patient Minimal	
99212	OF--Established Patient Low	
99213	OF--Established Patient Detailed	
99214	OF--Established Patient Moderate	X
99215	OF--Established Patient High	
PREVENTIVE VISITS - NEW		
99381	Under 1 Year	
99382	1 - 4 Years	
99383	5 - 11 Years	
99384	12 - 17 Years	
99385	18 - 39 Years	
99386	40 - 64 Years	
99387	65 Years & Up	
PREVENTIVE VISITS - ESTABLISHED		
99391	Under 1 Year	
99392	1 - 4 Years	
99393	5 - 11 Years	
99394	12 - 17 Years	
99395	18 - 39 Years	
99396	40 - 64 Years	
99397	65 Years & Up	
HOSPITAL/NURSING HOME VISITS		
99221	Initial hospital care, det.	
99222	Initial hospital care, comp.	
99223	Initial hospital care, high	
99281	ER Visit, min.	
99282	ER Visit, low	
99283	ER Visit, det.	
99284	ER Visit, moderate	
99285	ER Visit, high	
99307	Subseq. nursing facility care, pf.	

PROCEDURES		
10060	Incision/drainage, abcess	
20610	Aspiration, bursa	
29505	Splint, long leg	
29515	Splint, short leg	
36415	Routine venipuncture	
45330	Sigmoidoscopy, flex	
46600	Anoscopy, diagnostic	X
71030	Chest x-ray, complete	
73610	Radiology, ankle, complete	
93000	Routine ECG	
93018	Cardiovascular stress test	
99070	Supplies and materials	
LABORATORY		
80050	General health panel	
81000	Urinalysis, complete	
82270	Blood, occult, feces screening	X
82607	Vitamin B-12 test	
82948	Glucose, blood reagent	
85027	CBC, automated	
85651	Sedimentation rate test, manual	
86360	Absolute CD4/CD8 ratio	
86592	Syphilis test	
87070	Throat culture	
87088	Urine culture	
88150	Cytopathology, cervical or vaginal	
INJECTIONS		
90471	Immunization administration	
90472	Immunization administration, 2nd	
90658	Influenza injection, ages >3	
90702	DT immunization, ages <7	
90703	Tetanus immunization	
90707	MMR immunization	
90722	Therapeutic injection	
90723	DtaP - HepB - IPV	
90732	Pneumococcal immunization	

POLARIS MEDICAL GROUP

		NOTES
REFERRING PHYSICIAN	NPI	
AUTHORIZATION #		
DIAGNOSIS		
455.5		
PAYMENT AMOUNT		

Ohio Insurance Company
1600 Galleria Way
Cleveland, OH 44000

Polaris Medical Group
2100 Grace Avenue
Columbus, OH 43214

Practice ID: 09-012345

Date Prepared: 6/14/10

EFT Number: 0164297

Patient's Name	Dates of Service From - Thru	POS	Proc	Qty	Charge Amount	Allowed Amount	Patient Resp.	Amt. Paid Provider
Ferrara, Victoria	5/11/10 - 5/11/10	11	99212	1	$54.00	$54.00	$5.40	$48.60
Kavanaugh, Gregory	4/15/10 - 4/15/10	11	99213	1	$72.00	$72.00	$7.20	$64.80
Totals					$126.00	$126.00	$12.60	$113.40

* * * * * * * *   *EFT transmitted in the amount of $113.40*   * * * * * * * *

ENCOUNTER FORM

6/15/2010 11:30am	Dr. Michael Mahabir
DATE TIME	PROVIDER
Alan J. Harcar	HARCAAL0
PATIENT NAME	CHART #

OFFICE VISITS - SYMPTOMATIC - NEW		
99201	OF--New Patient Minimal	
99202	OF--New Patient Low	
99203	OF--New Patient Detailed	
99204	OF--New Patient Moderate	
99205	OF--New Patient High	
OFFICE VISITS - SYMPTOMATIC - ESTABLISHED		
99211	OF--Established Patient Minimal	
99212	OF--Established Patient Low	X
99213	OF--Established Patient Detailed	
99214	OF--Established Patient Moderate	
99215	OF--Established Patient High	
PREVENTIVE VISITS - NEW		
99381	Under 1 Year	
99382	1 - 4 Years	
99383	5 - 11 Years	
99384	12 - 17 Years	
99385	18 - 39 Years	
99386	40 - 64 Years	
99387	65 Years & Up	
PREVENTIVE VISITS - ESTABLISHED		
99391	Under 1 Year	
99392	1 - 4 Years	
99393	5 - 11 Years	
99394	12 - 17 Years	
99395	18 - 39 Years	
99396	40 - 64 Years	
99397	65 Years & Up	
HOSPITAL/NURSING HOME VISITS		
99221	Initial hospital care, det.	
99222	Initial hospital care, comp.	
99223	Initial hospital care, high	
99281	ER Visit, min.	
99282	ER Visit, low	
99283	ER Visit, det.	
99284	ER Visit, moderate	
99285	ER Visit, high	
99307	Subseq. nursing facility care, pf.	

PROCEDURES		
10060	Incision/drainage, abcess	
20610	Aspiration, bursa	
29505	Splint, long leg	
29515	Splint, short leg	
36415	Routine venipuncture	
45330	Sigmoidoscopy, flex	
46600	Anoscopy, diagnostic	
71030	Chest x-ray, complete	
73610	Radiology, ankle, complete	
93000	Routine ECG	
93018	Cardiovascular stress test	
99070	Supplies and materials	
LABORATORY		
80050	General health panel	
81000	Urinalysis, complete	
82270	Blood, occult, feces screening	
82607	Vitamin B-12 test	
82948	Glucose, blood reagent	
85027	CBC, automated	
85651	Sedimentation rate test, manual	
86360	Absolute CD4/CD8 ratio	
86592	Syphilis test	
87070	Throat culture	
87088	Urine culture	
88150	Cytopathology, cervical or vaginal	
INJECTIONS		
90471	Immunization administration	
90472	Immunization administration, 2nd	
90658	Influenza injection, ages >3	
90702	DT immunization, ages <7	
90703	Tetanus immunization	
90707	MMR immunization	
90722	Therapeutic injection	
90723	DtaP - HepB - IPV	
90732	Pneumococcal immunization	

POLARIS MEDICAL GROUP

		NOTES
REFERRING PHYSICIAN	NPI	
AUTHORIZATION #		
DIAGNOSIS 487.1		
PAYMENT AMOUNT $18.00 copay, check #1201		

PATIENT INFORMATION FORM

THIS SECTION REFERS TO PATIENT ONLY

Name: Nora B. McAniff	**Sex:** F	**Marital Status:** ☐S ☒M ☐D ☐W	**Birth Date:** 5/1/45

Address: 2300 First Avenue, Apt. D-40   **SS#:** 504-00-6758

City: Jackson   **State:** OH   **Zip:** 45640   **Employer:** Argene Interiors (part-time)   **Phone:**

Home Phone: 999-555-2309   **Employer's Address:** 1700 Watertown Avenue

Work Phone: 999-555-6978   **City:** Jackson   **State:** OH   **Zip:** 45640

Spouse's Name: John McAniff   **Spouse's Employer:** Town of Jackson

Emergency Contact: John McAniff   **Relationship:** Husband   **Phone #:** 999-555-1022

FILL IN IF PATIENT IS A MINOR

Parent/Guardian's Name: **Sex:**   **Marital Status:** ☐S ☐M ☐D ☐W   **Birth Date:**

Phone: **SS#:**

Address: **Employer:**   **Phone:**

City: **State:** **Zip:**   **Employer's Address:**

Student Status: **City:** **State:** **Zip:**

INSURANCE INFORMATION

Primary Insurance Company: Nationwide Medicare HMO   **Secondary Insurance Company:**

Subscriber's Name: Nora B. McAniff   **Birth Date:** 5/1/45   **Subscriber's Name:**   **Birth Date:**

Plan: HMO   **SS#:** 504-00-6758   **Plan:**

Policy #: 504-00-6758BSA   **Group #:**   **Policy #:**   **Group #:**

Copayment/Deductible: $5 copay   **Price Code:** A

OTHER INFORMATION

Reason for visit: stomach pain   **Allergy to Medication (list):**

Name of referring physician: **If auto accident, list date and state in which it occurred:**

I authorize treatment and agree to pay all fees and charges for the person named above. I agree to pay all charges shown by statements, promptly upon their presentation, unless credit arrangements are agreed upon in writing.

I authorize payment directly to POLARIS MEDICAL GROUP of insurance benefits otherwise payable to me. I hereby authorize the release of any medical information necessary in order to process a claim for payment in my behalf.

Nora B. McAniff   6/16/10

(Patient's Signature/Parent or Guardian's Signature)   (Date)

I plan to make payment of my medical expenses as follows (check one or more):

_____ Insurance (as above)   _X_ Cash/Check/Credit/Debit Card   _X_ Medicare   _____ Medicaid   _____ Workers' Comp.

ENCOUNTER FORM

6/16/2010 9:00am	Dr. Michael Mahabir
DATE TIME	PROVIDER
Nora B. McAniff	**MCANINO0**
PATIENT NAME	CHART #

OFFICE VISITS - SYMPTOMATIC - NEW		
99201	OF--New Patient Minimal	
99202	OF--New Patient Low	X
99203	OF--New Patient Detailed	
99204	OF--New Patient Moderate	
99205	OF--New Patient High	

OFFICE VISITS - SYMPTOMATIC - ESTABLISHED		
99211	OF--Established Patient Minimal	
99212	OF--Established Patient Low	
99213	OF--Established Patient Detailed	
99214	OF--Established Patient Moderate	
99215	OF--Established Patient High	

PREVENTIVE VISITS - NEW		
99381	Under 1 Year	
99382	1 - 4 Years	
99383	5 - 11 Years	
99384	12 - 17 Years	
99385	18 - 39 Years	
99386	40 - 64 Years	
99387	65 Years & Up	

PREVENTIVE VISITS - ESTABLISHED		
99391	Under 1 Year	
99392	1 - 4 Years	
99393	5 - 11 Years	
99394	12 - 17 Years	
99395	18 - 39 Years	
99396	40 - 64 Years	
99397	65 Years & Up	

HOSPITAL/NURSING HOME VISITS		
99221	Initial hospital care, det.	
99222	Initial hospital care, comp.	
99223	Initial hospital care, high	
99281	ER Visit, min.	
99282	ER Visit, low	
99283	ER Visit, det.	
99284	ER Visit, moderate	
99285	ER Visit, high	
99307	Subseq. nursing facility care, pf.	

PROCEDURES		
10060	Incision/drainage, abcess	
20610	Aspiration, bursa	
29505	Splint, long leg	
29515	Splint, short leg	
36415	Routine venipuncture	
45330	Sigmoidoscopy, flex	
46600	Anoscopy, diagnostic	
71030	Chest x-ray, complete	
73610	Radiology, ankle, complete	
93000	Routine ECG	
93018	Cardiovascular stress test	
99070	Supplies and materials	

LABORATORY		
80050	General health panel	
81000	Urinalysis, complete	
82270	Blood, occult, feces screening	
82607	Vitamin B-12 test	
82948	Glucose, blood reagent	
85027	CBC, automated	
85651	Sedimentation rate test, manual	
86360	Absolute CD4/CD8 ratio	
86592	Syphilis test	
87070	Throat culture	
87088	Urine culture	
88150	Cytopathology, cervical or vaginal	

INJECTIONS		
90471	Immunization administration	
90472	Immunization administration, 2nd	
90658	Influenza injection, ages >3	
90702	DT immunization, ages <7	
90703	Tetanus immunization	
90707	MMR immunization	
90722	Therapeutic injection	
90723	DtaP - HepB - IPV	
90732	Pneumococcal immunization	

POLARIS MEDICAL GROUP

		NOTES
REFERRING PHYSICIAN	NPI	
AUTHORIZATION #		
DIAGNOSIS 530.11		
PAYMENT AMOUNT $5.00 copay, check #984		

Blue Cross Blue Shield of Ohio
5000 First Street
Worthington, OH 43085

Polaris Medical Group
2100 Grace Avenue
Columbus, OH 43214

Practice ID: 04-5678901

Date Prepared: 6/14/10   EFT Number: 123896362

Patient's Name	Dates of Service From - Thru	POS	Proc	Qty	Charge Amount	Allowed Amount	Patient Resp.	Amt. Paid Provider
O'Keefe, Diana	5/19/10 - 5/19/10	11	99211	1	$36.00	$36.00	$10.80	$25.20
O'Keefe, Diana	5/19/10 - 5/19/10	11	85651	1	$24.00	$24.00	$7.20	$16.80
Totals					$60.00	$60.00	$18.00	$42.00

* * * * * * *   *EFT transmitted in the amount of $42.00*   * * * * * * *

Physician's Notes

Stewart Weintraub - Hospital Visit 6/16/10

ICD: 812.20

CPT: 99283

Nationwide Medicare
P.O. Box 7000
Columbus, OH 43214

Polaris Medical Group
2100 Grace Avenue
Columbus, OH 43214

Practice ID: 10-123456

Date Prepared: 6/10/10   EFT Number: 3642987

Patient's Name	Dates of Service From - Thru	POS	Proc	Qty	Charge Amount	Allowed Amount	Patient Resp.	Amt. Paid Provider
Ahmadian, George	5/26/10 - 5/26/10	11	99385	1	$215.00	**A	$106.00	**A
Ahmadian, George	5/26/10 - 5/26/10	11	82948	1	$18.00	$8.00	$1.60	$6.40
Totals					$233.00	$8.00	$107.60	$6.40

**A This procedure is denied for this patient.

* * * * * * *   *EFT transmitted in the amount of $6.40*   * * * * * * *

ENCOUNTER FORM

5/26/2010	9:00am	Dr. Michael Mahabir
DATE	TIME	PROVIDER

George O. Ahmadian	AHMADGE0
PATIENT NAME	CHART #

OFFICE VISITS - SYMPTOMATIC - NEW		
99201	OF--New Patient Minimal	
99202	OF--New Patient Low	
99203	OF--New Patient Detailed	
99204	OF--New Patient Moderate	
99205	OF--New Patient High	
OFFICE VISITS - SYMPTOMATIC - ESTABLISHED		
99211	OF--Established Patient Minimal	
99212	OF--Established Patient Low	
99213	OF--Established Patient Detailed	X
99214	OF--Established Patient Moderate	
99215	OF--Established Patient High	
PREVENTIVE VISITS - NEW		
99381	Under 1 Year	
99382	1 - 4 Years	
99383	5 - 11 Years	
99384	12 - 17 Years	
99385	18 - 39 Years	
99386	40 - 64 Years	
99387	65 Years & Up	
PREVENTIVE VISITS - ESTABLISHED		
99391	Under 1 Year	
99392	1 - 4 Years	
99393	5 - 11 Years	
99394	12 - 17 Years	
99395	18 - 39 Years	
99396	40 - 64 Years	
99397	65 Years & Up	
HOSPITAL/NURSING HOME VISITS		
99221	Initial hospital care, det.	
99222	Initial hospital care, comp.	
99223	Initial hospital care, high	
99281	ER Visit, min.	
99282	ER Visit, low	
99283	ER Visit, det.	
99284	ER Visit, moderate	
99285	ER Visit, high	
99307	Subseq. nursing facility care, pf.	

PROCEDURES		
10060	Incision/drainage, abcess	
20610	Aspiration, bursa	
29505	Splint, long leg	
29515	Splint, short leg	
36415	Routine venipuncture	
45330	Sigmoidoscopy, flex	
46600	Anoscopy, diagnostic	
71030	Chest x-ray, complete	
73610	Radiology, ankle, complete	
93000	Routine ECG	
93018	Cardiovascular stress test	
99070	Supplies and materials	
LABORATORY		
80050	General health panel	
81000	Urinalysis, complete	
82270	Blood, occult, feces screening	
82607	Vitamin B-12 test	
82948	Glucose, blood reagent	X
85027	CBC, automated	
85651	Sedimentation rate test, manual	
86360	Absolute CD4/CD8 ratio	
86592	Syphilis test	
87070	Throat culture	
87088	Urine culture	
88150	Cytopathology, cervical or vaginal	
INJECTIONS		
90471	Immunization administration	
90472	Immunization administration, 2nd	
90658	Influenza injection, ages >3	
90702	DT immunization, ages <7	
90703	Tetanus immunization	
90707	MMR immunization	
90722	Therapeutic injection	
90723	DtaP - HepB - IPV	
90732	Pneumococcal immunization	

POLARIS MEDICAL GROUP

REFERRING PHYSICIAN	NPI	NOTES
AUTHORIZATION #		
DIAGNOSIS 250.00, 401.9		
PAYMENT AMOUNT		

ENCOUNTER FORM

6/16/2010	2:00pm	Dr. Robin Crebore
DATE	TIME	PROVIDER

Victoria A. Ferrara		FERRAVI0
PATIENT NAME		CHART #

OFFICE VISITS - SYMPTOMATIC - NEW		
99201	OF--New Patient Minimal	
99202	OF--New Patient Low	
99203	OF--New Patient Detailed	
99204	OF--New Patient Moderate	
99205	OF--New Patient High	
OFFICE VISITS - SYMPTOMATIC - ESTABLISHED		
99211	OF--Established Patient Minimal	
99212	OF--Established Patient Low	X
99213	OF--Established Patient Detailed	
99214	OF--Established Patient Moderate	
99215	OF--Established Patient High	
PREVENTIVE VISITS - NEW		
99381	Under 1 Year	
99382	1 - 4 Years	
99383	5 - 11 Years	
99384	12 - 17 Years	
99385	18 - 39 Years	
99386	40 - 64 Years	
99387	65 Years & Up	
PREVENTIVE VISITS - ESTABLISHED		
99391	Under 1 Year	
99392	1 - 4 Years	
99393	5 - 11 Years	
99394	12 - 17 Years	
99395	18 - 39 Years	
99396	40 - 64 Years	
99397	65 Years & Up	
HOSPITAL/NURSING HOME VISITS		
99221	Initial hospital care, det.	
99222	Initial hospital care, comp.	
99223	Initial hospital care, high	
99281	ER Visit, min.	
99282	ER Visit, low	
99283	ER Visit, det.	
99284	ER Visit, moderate	
99285	ER Visit, high	
99307	Subseq. nursing facility care, pf.	

PROCEDURES		
10060	Incision/drainage, abcess	
20610	Aspiration, bursa	
29505	Splint, long leg	
29515	Splint, short leg	
36415	Routine venipuncture	
45330	Sigmoidoscopy, flex	
46600	Anoscopy, diagnostic	
71030	Chest x-ray, complete	
73610	Radiology, ankle, complete	
93000	Routine ECG	
93018	Cardiovascular stress test	
99070	Supplies and materials	
LABORATORY		
80050	General health panel	
81000	Urinalysis, complete	
82270	Blood, occult, feces screening	
82607	Vitamin B-12 test	
82948	Glucose, blood reagent	
85027	CBC, automated	
85651	Sedimentation rate test, manual	
86360	Absolute CD4/CD8 ratio	
86592	Syphilis test	
87070	Throat culture	
87088	Urine culture	
88150	Cytopathology, cervical or vaginal	
INJECTIONS		
90471	Immunization administration	
90472	Immunization administration, 2nd	
90658	Influenza injection, ages >3	
90702	DT immunization, ages <7	
90703	Tetanus immunization	
90707	MMR immunization	
90722	Therapeutic injection	
90723	DtaP - HepB - IPV	
90732	Pneumococcal immunization	

POLARIS MEDICAL GROUP

REFERRING PHYSICIAN	NPI	NOTES
AUTHORIZATION #		
DIAGNOSIS 879.8		
PAYMENT AMOUNT		

Preliminary information on Dr. Sylvia Serto, 6/16/2010

Sylvia T. Serto, M.D., F.A.C.P.

Polaris Medical Group

2100 Grace Avenue

Columbus, OH 43214

Phone: 999 555-9800

Fax: 999 555-9801

Specialty: Internal Medicine

Taxonomy Code: 207R00000X

Dr. Serto accepts assignment for Medicare and Medicaid (signature date: 1/1/2010).

License Number: 86-5991

EIN: 22-7294401

NPI: 1287654321

Medicare PIN: 22105488-12

Group Number: RM1234

Standard Health Care
1500 Summit Avenue, Suite 500
Cincinnati, OH 45000

Polaris Medical Group
2100 Grace Avenue
Columbus, OH 43214

Practice ID: 01-234567

Date Prepared: 6/15/10   EFT Number: 0347869

Patient's Name	Dates of Service From - Thru	POS	Proc	Qty	Charge Amount	Allowed Amount	Patient Resp.	Amt. Paid Provider
Rennagel, Marilyn	5/11/10 - 5/11/10	11	99213	1	$72.00	$62.00	$15.00	$47.00
Rennagel, Marilyn	5/11/10 - 5/11/10	11	81000	1	$22.00	$17.00	$0.00	$17.00
Rennagel, Marilyn	5/11/10 - 5/11/10	11	82948	1	$18.00	$15.00	$0.00	$15.00
Totals					$112.00	$94.00	$15.00	$79.00

* * * * * * * *   *EFT transmitted in the amount of $79.00*   * * * * * * * *

PATIENT INFORMATION FORM

THIS SECTION REFERS TO PATIENT ONLY

Name: Angelo X. Daiute	Sex: M	Marital Status: ☐ S ☒ M ☐ D ☐ W	Birth Date: 1/5/70

Address: 22 Van Cortland Drive, Apt. 390	SS#: 756-99-2637		

City: Fairview	State: OH	Zip: 43773	Employer: COSTINC (full-time)	Phone:

Home Phone: 999-555-1758	Employer's Address: 3504 Overland Avenue		

Work Phone: 999-555-4300	City: Columbus	State: OH	Zip: 43214

Spouse's Name: Mary Daiute	Spouse's Employer: not employed

Emergency Contact: Mary Daiute	Relationship: wife	Phone #: 999-555-1758

FILL IN IF PATIENT IS A MINOR

Parent/Guardian's Name:	Sex:	Marital Status: ☐ S ☐ M ☐ D ☐ W	Birth Date:

Phone:	SS#:

Address:	Employer:	Phone:

City:	State:	Zip:	Employer's Address:

Student Status:	City:	State:	Zip:

INSURANCE INFORMATION

Primary Insurance Company: Standard Health Care	Secondary Insurance Company:

Subscriber's Name: Angelo X. Daiute	Birth Date: 1/5/70	Subscriber's Name:	Birth Date:

Plan: PPO	SS#: 756-99-2637	Plan:

Policy #: 000-AD9876	Group #: CSTAA	Policy #:	Group #:

Copayment/Deductible: $15 / $1,000	Price Code: A	

OTHER INFORMATION

Reason for visit: comprehensive physical examination	Allergy to Medication (list):

Name of referring physician:	If auto accident, list date and state in which it occurred:

I authorize treatment and agree to pay all fees and charges for the person named above. I agree to pay all charges shown by statements, promptly upon their presentation, unless credit arrangements are agreed upon in writing.

I authorize payment directly to POLARIS MEDICAL GROUP of insurance benefits otherwise payable to me. I hereby authorize the release of any medical information necessary in order to process a claim for payment in my behalf.

Angelo X. Daiute	6/17/10
(Patient's Signature/Parent or Guardian's Signature)	(Date)

I plan to make payment of my medical expenses as follows (check one or more):

__X__ Insurance (as above)　　__X__ Cash/Check/Credit/Debit Card　　_____ Medicare　　_____ Medicaid　　_____ Workers' Comp.

ENCOUNTER FORM

6/17/2010 10:30am	Dr. Robin Crebore
DATE TIME	PROVIDER
Angelo X. Daiute	DAIUTAN0
PATIENT NAME	CHART #

OFFICE VISITS - SYMPTOMATIC - NEW		
99201	OF--New Patient Minimal	
99202	OF--New Patient Low	
99203	OF--New Patient Detailed	
99204	OF--New Patient Moderate	
99205	OF--New Patient High	
OFFICE VISITS - SYMPTOMATIC - ESTABLISHED		
99211	OF--Established Patient Minimal	
99212	OF--Established Patient Low	
99213	OF--Established Patient Detailed	
99214	OF--Established Patient Moderate	
99215	OF--Established Patient High	
PREVENTIVE VISITS - NEW		
99381	Under 1 Year	
99382	1 - 4 Years	
99383	5 - 11 Years	
99384	12 - 17 Years	
99385	18 - 39 Years	
99386	40 - 64 Years	X
99387	65 Years & Up	
PREVENTIVE VISITS - ESTABLISHED		
99391	Under 1 Year	
99392	1 - 4 Years	
99393	5 - 11 Years	
99394	12 - 17 Years	
99395	18 - 39 Years	
99396	40 - 64 Years	
99397	65 Years & Up	
HOSPITAL/NURSING HOME VISITS		
99221	Initial hospital care, det.	
99222	Initial hospital care, comp.	
99223	Initial hospital care, high	
99281	ER Visit, min.	
99282	ER Visit, low	
99283	ER Visit, det.	
99284	ER Visit, moderate	
99285	ER Visit, high	
99307	Subseq. nursing facility care, pf.	

PROCEDURES		
10060	Incision/drainage, abcess	
20610	Aspiration, bursa	
29505	Splint, long leg	
29515	Splint, short leg	
36415	Routine venipuncture	X
45330	Sigmoidoscopy, flex	
46600	Anoscopy, diagnostic	
71030	Chest x-ray, complete	
73610	Radiology, ankle, complete	
93000	Routine ECG	X
93018	Cardiovascular stress test	
99070	Supplies and materials	
LABORATORY		
80050	General health panel	X
81000	Urinalysis, complete	X
82270	Blood, occult, feces screening	
82607	Vitamin B-12 test	
82948	Glucose, blood reagent	
85027	CBC, automated	
85651	Sedimentation rate test, manual	
86360	Absolute CD4/CD8 ratio	
86592	Syphilis test	
87070	Throat culture	
87088	Urine culture	
88150	Cytopathology, cervical or vaginal	
INJECTIONS		
90471	Immunization administration	
90472	Immunization administration, 2nd	
90658	Influenza injection, ages >3	
90702	DT immunization, ages <7	
90703	Tetanus immunization	
90707	MMR immunization	
90722	Therapeutic injection	
90723	DtaP - HepB - IPV	
90732	Pneumococcal immunization	

POLARIS MEDICAL GROUP		NOTES
REFERRING PHYSICIAN	NPI	
AUTHORIZATION #		
DIAGNOSIS v70.0		
PAYMENT AMOUNT $15.00 copay, check #3317		

ENCOUNTER FORM

6/17/2010   2:00pm
DATE   TIME

Dr. Michael Mahabir
PROVIDER

Cameron T. Trotta
PATIENT NAME

TROTTCA0
CHART #

OFFICE VISITS - SYMPTOMATIC - NEW		
99201	OF--New Patient Minimal	
99202	OF--New Patient Low	
99203	OF--New Patient Detailed	
99204	OF--New Patient Moderate	
99205	OF--New Patient High	
OFFICE VISITS - SYMPTOMATIC - ESTABLISHED		
99211	OF--Established Patient Minimal	
99212	OF--Established Patient Low	
99213	OF--Established Patient Detailed	
99214	OF--Established Patient Moderate	
99215	OF--Established Patient High	
PREVENTIVE VISITS - NEW		
99381	Under 1 Year	
99382	1 - 4 Years	
99383	5 - 11 Years	
99384	12 - 17 Years	
99385	18 - 39 Years	
99386	40 - 64 Years	
99387	65 Years & Up	
PREVENTIVE VISITS - ESTABLISHED		
99391	Under 1 Year	
99392	1 - 4 Years	
99393	5 - 11 Years	
99394	12 - 17 Years	
99395	18 - 39 Years	
99396	40 - 64 Years	X
99397	65 Years & Up	
HOSPITAL/NURSING HOME VISITS		
99221	Initial hospital care, det.	
99222	Initial hospital care, comp.	
99223	Initial hospital care, high	
99281	ER Visit, min.	
99282	ER Visit, low	
99283	ER Visit, det.	
99284	ER Visit, moderate	
99285	ER Visit, high	
99307	Subseq. nursing facility care, pf.	

PROCEDURES		
10060	Incision/drainage, abscess	
20610	Aspiration, bursa	
29505	Splint, long leg	
29515	Splint, short leg	
36415	Routine venipuncture	X
45330	Sigmoidoscopy, flex	
46600	Anoscopy, diagnostic	
71030	Chest x-ray, complete	
73610	Radiology, ankle, complete	
93000	Routine ECG	X
93018	Cardiovascular stress test	
99070	Supplies and materials	
LABORATORY		
80050	General health panel	X
81000	Urinalysis, complete	X
82270	Blood, occult, feces screening	X
82607	Vitamin B-12 test	
82948	Glucose, blood reagent	
85027	CBC, automated	
85651	Sedimentation rate test, manual	
86360	Absolute CD4/CD8 ratio	
86592	Syphilis test	
87070	Throat culture	
87088	Urine culture	
88150	Cytopathology, cervical or vaginal	
INJECTIONS		
90471	Immunization administration	
90472	Immunization administration, 2nd	
90658	Influenza injection, ages >3	
90702	DT immunization, ages <7	
90703	Tetanus immunization	
90707	MMR immunization	
90722	Therapeutic injection	
90723	DtaP - HepB - IPV	
90732	Pneumococcal immunization	

POLARIS MEDICAL GROUP

REFERRING PHYSICIAN

NPI

NOTES

AUTHORIZATION #

DIAGNOSIS
v70.0

PAYMENT AMOUNT
$18.00 copay, check #869

ENCOUNTER FORM

6/17/2010 **3:00pm** DATE TIME	**Dr. Michael Mahabir** PROVIDER
George O. Ahmadian PATIENT NAME	**AHMADGE0** CHART #

OFFICE VISITS - SYMPTOMATIC - NEW		
99201	OF--New Patient Minimal	
99202	OF--New Patient Low	
99203	OF--New Patient Detailed	
99204	OF--New Patient Moderate	
99205	OF--New Patient High	

OFFICE VISITS - SYMPTOMATIC - ESTABLISHED		
99211	OF--Established Patient Minimal	
99212	OF--Established Patient Low	
99213	OF--Established Patient Detailed	
99214	OF--Established Patient Moderate	
99215	OF--Established Patient High	X

PREVENTIVE VISITS - NEW		
99381	Under 1 Year	
99382	1 - 4 Years	
99383	5 - 11 Years	
99384	12 - 17 Years	
99385	18 - 39 Years	
99386	40 - 64 Years	
99387	65 Years & Up	

PREVENTIVE VISITS - ESTABLISHED		
99391	Under 1 Year	
99392	1 - 4 Years	
99393	5 - 11 Years	
99394	12 - 17 Years	
99395	18 - 39 Years	
99396	40 - 64 Years	
99397	65 Years & Up	

HOSPITAL/NURSING HOME VISITS		
99221	Initial hospital care, det.	
99222	Initial hospital care, comp.	
99223	Initial hospital care, high	
99281	ER Visit, min.	
99282	ER Visit, low	
99283	ER Visit, det.	
99284	ER Visit, moderate	
99285	ER Visit, high	
99307	Subseq. nursing facility care, pf.	

PROCEDURES		
10060	Incision/drainage, abcess	
20610	Aspiration, bursa	
29505	Splint, long leg	
29515	Splint, short leg	
36415	Routine venipuncture	
45330	Sigmoidoscopy, flex	
46600	Anoscopy, diagnostic	
71030	Chest x-ray, complete	
73610	Radiology, ankle, complete	
93000	Routine ECG	
93018	Cardiovascular stress test	
99070	Supplies and materials	

LABORATORY		
80050	General health panel	
81000	Urinalysis, complete	
82270	Blood, occult, feces screening	
82607	Vitamin B-12 test	
82948	Glucose, blood reagent	
85027	CBC, automated	
85651	Sedimentation rate test, manual	
86360	Absolute CD4/CD8 ratio	
86592	Syphilis test	
87070	Throat culture	
87088	Urine culture	
88150	Cytopathology, cervical or vaginal	

INJECTIONS		
90471	Immunization administration	
90472	Immunization administration, 2nd	
90658	Influenza injection, ages >3	
90702	DT immunization, ages <7	
90703	Tetanus immunization	
90707	MMR immunization	
90722	Therapeutic injection	
90723	DtaP - HepB - IPV	
90732	Pneumococcal immunization	

POLARIS MEDICAL GROUP

			NOTES
REFERRING PHYSICIAN		NPI	
AUTHORIZATION #			
DIAGNOSIS **331.0**			
PAYMENT AMOUNT			

Standard Health Care
1500 Summit Avenue, Suite 500
Cincinnati, OH 45000

Polaris Medical Group
2100 Grace Avenue
Columbus, OH 43214

Practice ID: 01-234567

Date Prepared: 6/16/10

EFT Number: 035102

Patient's Name	Dates of Service From - Thru	POS	Proc	Qty	Charge Amount	Allowed Amount	Patient Resp.	Amt. Paid Provider
Szinovacz, Martin G	5/27/10 - 5/27/10	11	99395	1	$178.00	$137.00	$15.00	$122.00
Szinovacz, Martin G	5/27/10 - 5/27/10	11	36415	1	$22.00	$17.00	$0.00	$17.00
Szinovacz, Martin G	5/27/10 - 5/27/10	11	80050	1	$143.00	$120.00	$0.00	$120.00
Szinovacz, Martin G	5/27/10 - 5/27/10	11	81000	1	$22.00	$17.00	$0.00	$17.00
Szinovacz, Martin G	5/27/10 - 5/27/10	11	93000	1	$84.00	$70.00	$0.00	$70.00

| Totals | | | | | $449.00 | $361.00 | $15.00 | $346.00 |

* * * * * * * *   *EFT transmitted in the amount of $346.00*   * * * * * * * *

PATIENT INFORMATION FORM

THIS SECTION REFERS TO PATIENT ONLY

Name: Hector M. Valaquez			Sex: M	Marital Status: ☐ S ☒ M ☐ D ☐ W	Birth Date: 8/15/82

Address: 199 Transfer Street			SS#: 459-94-9934	

City: Highland	State: OH	Zip: 45132	Employer: COSTINC (full-time)	Phone:

Home Phone: 999-555-3364	Employer's Address: 3504 Overland Avenue

Work Phone: 999-555-3867	City: Columbus	State: OH	Zip: 43214

Spouse's Name: Juanita T. Valaquez	Spouse's Employer: Hapgood School District

Emergency Contact: Juanita T. Valaquez	Relationship: wife	Phone #: 999-555-3364

FILL IN IF PATIENT IS A MINOR

Parent/Guardian's Name:	Sex:	Marital Status: ☐ S ☐ M ☐ D ☐ W	Birth Date:

Phone:	SS#:

Address:	Employer:	Phone:

City:	State:	Zip:	Employer's Address:

Student Status:	City:	State:	Zip:

INSURANCE INFORMATION

Primary Insurance Company: Aetna Health Plans	Secondary Insurance Company:

Subscriber's Name: Hector M. Valaquez	Birth Date: 8/15/82	Subscriber's Name:	Birth Date:

Plan: Ohio HMO	SS#: 459-94-9934	Plan:

Policy #: 134GG	Group #: COS 41	Policy #:	Group #:

Copayment/Deductible: $15 copay	Price Code: A	

OTHER INFORMATION

Reason for visit: sunburn	Allergy to Medication (list):

Name of referring physician:	If auto accident, list date and state in which it occurred:

I authorize treatment and agree to pay all fees and charges for the person named above. I agree to pay all charges shown by statements, promptly upon their presentation, unless credit arrangements are agreed upon in writing.

I authorize payment directly to POLARIS MEDICAL GROUP of insurance benefits otherwise payable to me. I hereby authorize the release of any medical information necessary in order to process a claim for payment in my behalf.

Hector M. Valaquez	6/18/10
(Patient's Signature/Parent or Guardian's Signature)	(Date)

I plan to make payment of my medical expenses as follows (check one or more):

__X__ Insurance (as above)   __X__ Cash/Check/Credit/Debit Card   _____ Medicare   _____ Medicaid   _____ Workers' Comp.

ENCOUNTER FORM

__6/18/2010__   __9:00am__   __Dr. Robin Crebore__
DATE   TIME   PROVIDER

__Hector M. Valaquez__   __VALAQHE0__
PATIENT NAME   CHART #

OFFICE VISITS - SYMPTOMATIC - NEW		
99201	OF--New Patient Minimal	X
99202	OF--New Patient Low	
99203	OF--New Patient Detailed	
99204	OF--New Patient Moderate	
99205	OF--New Patient High	
OFFICE VISITS - SYMPTOMATIC - ESTABLISHED		
99211	OF--Established Patient Minimal	
99212	OF--Established Patient Low	
99213	OF--Established Patient Detailed	
99214	OF--Established Patient Moderate	
99215	OF--Established Patient High	
PREVENTIVE VISITS - NEW		
99381	Under 1 Year	
99382	1 - 4 Years	
99383	5 - 11 Years	
99384	12 - 17 Years	
99385	18 - 39 Years	
99386	40 - 64 Years	
99387	65 Years & Up	
PREVENTIVE VISITS - ESTABLISHED		
99391	Under 1 Year	
99392	1 - 4 Years	
99393	5 - 11 Years	
99394	12 - 17 Years	
99395	18 - 39 Years	
99396	40 - 64 Years	
99397	65 Years & Up	
HOSPITAL/NURSING HOME VISITS		
99221	Initial hospital care, det.	
99222	Initial hospital care, comp.	
99223	Initial hospital care, high	
99281	ER Visit, min.	
99282	ER Visit, low	
99283	ER Visit, det.	
99284	ER Visit, moderate	
99285	ER Visit, high	
99307	Subseq. nursing facility care, pf.	

PROCEDURES		
10060	Incision/drainage, abcess	
20610	Aspiration, bursa	
29505	Splint, long leg	
29515	Splint, short leg	
36415	Routine venipuncture	
45330	Sigmoidoscopy, flex	
46600	Anoscopy, diagnostic	
71030	Chest x-ray, complete	
73610	Radiology, ankle, complete	
93000	Routine ECG	
93018	Cardiovascular stress test	
99070	Supplies and materials	
LABORATORY		
80050	General health panel	
81000	Urinalysis, complete	
82270	Blood, occult, feces screening	
82607	Vitamin B-12 test	
82948	Glucose, blood reagent	
85027	CBC, automated	
85651	Sedimentation rate test, manual	
86360	Absolute CD4/CD8 ratio	
86592	Syphilis test	
87070	Throat culture	
87088	Urine culture	
88150	Cytopathology, cervical or vaginal	
INJECTIONS		
90471	Immunization administration	
90472	Immunization administration, 2nd	
90658	Influenza injection, ages >3	
90702	DT immunization, ages <7	
90703	Tetanus immunization	
90707	MMR immunization	
90722	Therapeutic injection	
90723	DtaP - HepB - IPV	
90732	Pneumococcal immunization	

POLARIS MEDICAL GROUP

NOTES

REFERRING PHYSICIAN   NPI

AUTHORIZATION #

DIAGNOSIS
__692.71__

PAYMENT AMOUNT
 $15.00 copay, check #3231

ENCOUNTER FORM

6/18/2010	9:30am	Dr. Robin Crebore
DATE	TIME	PROVIDER
Seymour B. Colbs		COLBSSE0
PATIENT NAME		CHART #

OFFICE VISITS - SYMPTOMATIC - NEW		
99201	OF--New Patient Minimal	
99202	OF--New Patient Low	
99203	OF--New Patient Detailed	
99204	OF--New Patient Moderate	
99205	OF--New Patient High	
OFFICE VISITS - SYMPTOMATIC - ESTABLISHED		
99211	OF--Established Patient Minimal	
99212	OF--Established Patient Low	
99213	OF--Established Patient Detailed	X
99214	OF--Established Patient Moderate	
99215	OF--Established Patient High	
PREVENTIVE VISITS - NEW		
99381	Under 1 Year	
99382	1 - 4 Years	
99383	5 - 11 Years	
99384	12 - 17 Years	
99385	18 - 39 Years	
99386	40 - 64 Years	
99387	65 Years & Up	
PREVENTIVE VISITS - ESTABLISHED		
99391	Under 1 Year	
99392	1 - 4 Years	
99393	5 - 11 Years	
99394	12 - 17 Years	
99395	18 - 39 Years	
99396	40 - 64 Years	
99397	65 Years & Up	
HOSPITAL/NURSING HOME VISITS		
99221	Initial hospital care, det.	
99222	Initial hospital care, comp.	
99223	Initial hospital care, high	
99281	ER Visit, min.	
99282	ER Visit, low	
99283	ER Visit, det.	
99284	ER Visit, moderate	
99285	ER Visit, high	
99307	Subseq. nursing facility care, pf.	

PROCEDURES		
10060	Incision/drainage, abcess	
20610	Aspiration, bursa	
29505	Splint, long leg	
29515	Splint, short leg	
36415	Routine venipuncture	
45330	Sigmoidoscopy, flex	
46600	Anoscopy, diagnostic	
71030	Chest x-ray, complete	
73610	Radiology, ankle, complete	
93000	Routine ECG	
93018	Cardiovascular stress test	
99070	Supplies and materials	
LABORATORY		
80050	General health panel	
81000	Urinalysis, complete	
82270	Blood, occult, feces screening	
82607	Vitamin B-12 test	
82948	Glucose, blood reagent	
85027	CBC, automated	
85651	Sedimentation rate test, manual	
86360	Absolute CD4/CD8 ratio	
86592	Syphilis test	
87070	Throat culture	
87088	Urine culture	
88150	Cytopathology, cervical or vaginal	
INJECTIONS		
90471	Immunization administration	
90472	Immunization administration, 2nd	
90658	Influenza injection, ages >3	
90702	DT immunization, ages <7	
90703	Tetanus immunization	
90707	MMR immunization	
90722	Therapeutic injection	
90723	DtaP - HepB - IPV	
90732	Pneumococcal immunization	

POLARIS MEDICAL GROUP

		NOTES
REFERRING PHYSICIAN	NPI	
AUTHORIZATION #		
DIAGNOSIS 882.0		
PAYMENT AMOUNT $8.25 copay, check #839		

ENCOUNTER FORM

6/18/2010 10:00am	Dr. Robin Crebore
DATE TIME	PROVIDER
David R. Weatherly	WEATHDA0
PATIENT NAME	CHART #

OFFICE VISITS - SYMPTOMATIC - NEW		
99201	OF--New Patient Minimal	
99202	OF--New Patient Low	
99203	OF--New Patient Detailed	
99204	OF--New Patient Moderate	
99205	OF--New Patient High	

OFFICE VISITS - SYMPTOMATIC - ESTABLISHED		
99211	OF--Established Patient Minimal	
99212	OF--Established Patient Low	
99213	OF--Established Patient Detailed	
99214	OF--Established Patient Moderate	X
99215	OF--Established Patient High	

PREVENTIVE VISITS - NEW		
99381	Under 1 Year	
99382	1 - 4 Years	
99383	5 - 11 Years	
99384	12 - 17 Years	
99385	18 - 39 Years	
99386	40 - 64 Years	
99387	65 Years & Up	

PREVENTIVE VISITS - ESTABLISHED		
99391	Under 1 Year	
99392	1 - 4 Years	
99393	5 - 11 Years	
99394	12 - 17 Years	
99395	18 - 39 Years	
99396	40 - 64 Years	
99397	65 Years & Up	

HOSPITAL/NURSING HOME VISITS		
99221	Initial hospital care, det.	
99222	Initial hospital care, comp.	
99223	Initial hospital care, high	
99281	ER Visit, min.	
99282	ER Visit, low	
99283	ER Visit, det.	
99284	ER Visit, moderate	
99285	ER Visit, high	
99307	Subseq. nursing facility care, pf.	

PROCEDURES		
10060	Incision/drainage, abcess	
20610	Aspiration, bursa	
29505	Splint, long leg	
29515	Splint, short leg	
36415	Routine venipuncture	
45330	Sigmoidoscopy, flex	
46600	Anoscopy, diagnostic	
71030	Chest x-ray, complete	X
73610	Radiology, ankle, complete	
93000	Routine ECG	X
93018	Cardiovascular stress test	
99070	Supplies and materials	

LABORATORY		
80050	General health panel	
81000	Urinalysis, complete	
82270	Blood, occult, feces screening	
82607	Vitamin B-12 test	
82948	Glucose, blood reagent	
85027	CBC, automated	
85651	Sedimentation rate test, manual	
86360	Absolute CD4/CD8 ratio	
86592	Syphilis test	
87070	Throat culture	
87088	Urine culture	
88150	Cytopathology, cervical or vaginal	

INJECTIONS		
90471	Immunization administration	
90472	Immunization administration, 2nd	
90658	Influenza injection, ages >3	
90702	DT immunization, ages <7	
90703	Tetanus immunization	
90707	MMR immunization	
90722	Therapeutic injection	
90723	DtaP - HepB - IPV	
90732	Pneumococcal immunization	

POLARIS MEDICAL GROUP

		NOTES
REFERRING PHYSICIAN	NPI	
AUTHORIZATION #		
DIAGNOSIS 493.00		
PAYMENT AMOUNT $18.00 copay, check #2312		

Electronic Claim Audit/Edit Report

Polaris Medical Group
2100 Grace Avenue
Columbus, OH 43214

Transmission Number: 6071298

Insurance Carrier: Medicare

Patient's Name	Dates of Service From - Thru	POS	Proc	Qty	Status
Atchely, Rachel	5/26/10 - 5/26/10	31	99202	1	Rejected**

** see reason for rejection below

********** *Incorrect procedure code* **********

ENCOUNTER FORM

6/18/2010   10:45am
DATE   TIME

Dr. Michael Mahabir
PROVIDER

Roberta Yange-Sang
PATIENT NAME

YANGERO0
CHART #

OFFICE VISITS - SYMPTOMATIC - NEW		
99201	OF--New Patient Minimal	
99202	OF--New Patient Low	
99203	OF--New Patient Detailed	
99204	OF--New Patient Moderate	
99205	OF--New Patient High	
OFFICE VISITS - SYMPTOMATIC - ESTABLISHED		
99211	OF--Established Patient Minimal	
99212	OF--Established Patient Low	X
99213	OF--Established Patient Detailed	
99214	OF--Established Patient Moderate	
99215	OF--Established Patient High	
PREVENTIVE VISITS - NEW		
99381	Under 1 Year	
99382	1 - 4 Years	
99383	5 - 11 Years	
99384	12 - 17 Years	
99385	18 - 39 Years	
99386	40 - 64 Years	
99387	65 Years & Up	
PREVENTIVE VISITS - ESTABLISHED		
99391	Under 1 Year	
99392	1 - 4 Years	
99393	5 - 11 Years	
99394	12 - 17 Years	
99395	18 - 39 Years	
99396	40 - 64 Years	
99397	65 Years & Up	
HOSPITAL/NURSING HOME VISITS		
99221	Initial hospital care, det.	
99222	Initial hospital care, comp.	
99223	Initial hospital care, high	
99281	ER Visit, min.	
99282	ER Visit, low	
99283	ER Visit, det.	
99284	ER Visit, moderate	
99285	ER Visit, high	
99307	Subseq. nursing facility care, pf.	

PROCEDURES		
10060	Incision/drainage, abcess	
20610	Aspiration, bursa	
29505	Splint, long leg	
29515	Splint, short leg	
36415	Routine venipuncture	
45330	Sigmoidoscopy, flex	
46600	Anoscopy, diagnostic	
71030	Chest x-ray, complete	
73610	Radiology, ankle, complete	
93000	Routine ECG	
93018	Cardiovascular stress test	
99070	Supplies and materials	
LABORATORY		
80050	General health panel	
81000	Urinalysis, complete	
82270	Blood, occult, feces screening	
82607	Vitamin B-12 test	
82948	Glucose, blood reagent	
85027	CBC, automated	
85651	Sedimentation rate test, manual	
86360	Absolute CD4/CD8 ratio	
86592	Syphilis test	
87070	Throat culture	
87088	Urine culture	
88150	Cytopathology, cervical or vaginal	
INJECTIONS		
90471	Immunization administration	
90472	Immunization administration, 2nd	
90658	Influenza injection, ages >3	
90702	DT immunization, ages <7	
90703	Tetanus immunization	
90707	MMR immunization	
90722	Therapeutic injection	
90723	DtaP - HepB - IPV	
90732	Pneumococcal immunization	

POLARIS MEDICAL GROUP

REFERRING PHYSICIAN

NPI

NOTES

AUTHORIZATION #

DIAGNOSIS
891.0

PAYMENT AMOUNT
$8.25 copay, check #240

ENCOUNTER FORM

6/18/2010 2:45pm	Dr. Michael Mahabir
DATE TIME	PROVIDER
Gloria Berkel-Rees	BERKEGL0
PATIENT NAME	CHART #

OFFICE VISITS - SYMPTOMATIC - NEW		
99201	OF--New Patient Minimal	
99202	OF--New Patient Low	
99203	OF--New Patient Detailed	
99204	OF--New Patient Moderate	
99205	OF--New Patient High	

OFFICE VISITS - SYMPTOMATIC - ESTABLISHED		
99211	OF--Established Patient Minimal	
99212	OF--Established Patient Low	
99213	OF--Established Patient Detailed	X
99214	OF--Established Patient Moderate	
99215	OF--Established Patient High	

PREVENTIVE VISITS - NEW		
99381	Under 1 Year	
99382	1 - 4 Years	
99383	5 - 11 Years	
99384	12 - 17 Years	
99385	18 - 39 Years	
99386	40 - 64 Years	
99387	65 Years & Up	

PREVENTIVE VISITS - ESTABLISHED		
99391	Under 1 Year	
99392	1 - 4 Years	
99393	5 - 11 Years	
99394	12 - 17 Years	
99395	18 - 39 Years	
99396	40 - 64 Years	
99397	65 Years & Up	

HOSPITAL/NURSING HOME VISITS		
99221	Initial hospital care, det.	
99222	Initial hospital care, comp.	
99223	Initial hospital care, high	
99281	ER Visit, min.	
99282	ER Visit, low	
99283	ER Visit, det.	
99284	ER Visit, moderate	
99285	ER Visit, high	
99307	Subseq. nursing facility care, pf.	

PROCEDURES		
10060	Incision/drainage, abcess	
20610	Aspiration, bursa	
29505	Splint, long leg	
29515	Splint, short leg	
36415	Routine venipuncture	
45330	Sigmoidoscopy, flex	
46600	Anoscopy, diagnostic	
71030	Chest x-ray, complete	
73610	Radiology, ankle, complete	
93000	Routine ECG	
93018	Cardiovascular stress test	
99070	Supplies and materials	X

LABORATORY		
80050	General health panel	
81000	Urinalysis, complete	
82270	Blood, occult, feces screening	
82607	Vitamin B-12 test	
82948	Glucose, blood reagent	
85027	CBC, automated	
85651	Sedimentation rate test, manual	
86360	Absolute CD4/CD8 ratio	
86592	Syphilis test	
87070	Throat culture	
87088	Urine culture	
88150	Cytopathology, cervical or vaginal	

INJECTIONS		
90471	Immunization administration	
90472	Immunization administration, 2nd	
90658	Influenza injection, ages >3	
90702	DT immunization, ages <7	
90703	Tetanus immunization	
90707	MMR immunization	
90722	Therapeutic injection	
90723	DtaP - HepB - IPV	
90732	Pneumococcal immunization	

POLARIS MEDICAL GROUP

REFERRING PHYSICIAN	NPI	NOTES
		99070 supplies and materials $15.00
AUTHORIZATION #		
DIAGNOSIS		
493.00		
PAYMENT AMOUNT		

ENCOUNTER FORM

6/18/2010 4:00pm	Dr. Michael Mahabir
DATE TIME	PROVIDER
Alan J. Harcar	HARCAAL0
PATIENT NAME	CHART #

OFFICE VISITS - SYMPTOMATIC - NEW

99201	OF--New Patient Minimal	
99202	OF--New Patient Low	
99203	OF--New Patient Detailed	
99204	OF--New Patient Moderate	
99205	OF--New Patient High	

OFFICE VISITS - SYMPTOMATIC - ESTABLISHED

99211	OF--Established Patient Minimal	
99212	OF--Established Patient Low	
99213	OF--Established Patient Detailed	
99214	OF--Established Patient Moderate	
99215	OF--Established Patient High	

PREVENTIVE VISITS - NEW

99381	Under 1 Year	
99382	1 - 4 Years	
99383	5 - 11 Years	
99384	12 - 17 Years	
99385	18 - 39 Years	
99386	40 - 64 Years	
99387	65 Years & Up	

PREVENTIVE VISITS - ESTABLISHED

99391	Under 1 Year	
99392	1 - 4 Years	
99393	5 - 11 Years	
99394	12 - 17 Years	
99395	18 - 39 Years	
99396	40 - 64 Years	
99397	65 Years & Up	X

HOSPITAL/NURSING HOME VISITS

99221	Initial hospital care, det.	
99222	Initial hospital care, comp.	
99223	Initial hospital care, high	
99281	ER Visit, min.	
99282	ER Visit, low	
99283	ER Visit, det.	
99284	ER Visit, moderate	
99285	ER Visit, high	
99307	Subseq. nursing facility care, pf.	

PROCEDURES

10060	Incision/drainage, abcess	
20610	Aspiration, bursa	
29505	Splint, long leg	
29515	Splint, short leg	
36415	Routine venipuncture	X
45330	Sigmoidoscopy, flex	
46600	Anoscopy, diagnostic	
71030	Chest x-ray, complete	
73610	Radiology, ankle, complete	
93000	Routine ECG	X
93018	Cardiovascular stress test	
99070	Supplies and materials	

LABORATORY

80050	General health panel	X
81000	Urinalysis, complete	X
82270	Blood, occult, feces screening	
82607	Vitamin B-12 test	
82948	Glucose, blood reagent	
85027	CBC, automated	
85651	Sedimentation rate test, manual	
86360	Absolute CD4/CD8 ratio	
86592	Syphilis test	
87070	Throat culture	
87088	Urine culture	
88150	Cytopathology, cervical or vaginal	

INJECTIONS

90471	Immunization administration	
90472	Immunization administration, 2nd	
90658	Influenza injection, ages >3	
90702	DT immunization, ages <7	
90703	Tetanus immunization	
90707	MMR immunization	
90722	Therapeutic injection	
90723	DtaP - HepB - IPV	
90732	Pneumococcal immunization	

POLARIS MEDICAL GROUP

		NOTES
REFERRING PHYSICIAN	NPI	
AUTHORIZATION #		
DIAGNOSIS v70.0		
PAYMENT AMOUNT $18.00 copay, check #1024		

Physician's Notes

Myrna Beedon - Hospital Visit 6/21/10

ICD: 746.9

CPT: 99222

PATIENT INFORMATION FORM

THIS SECTION REFERS TO PATIENT ONLY

Name: Fran C. Ferrone	Sex: F	Marital Status: ☐ S ☐ M ☒ D ☐ W	Birth Date: 3/30/50
Address: 1050 Southway	SS#: 332-75-9360		

City: Fairview	State: OH	Zip: 43773	Employer: Woodworkers Warehouse (full-time)	Phone: 999-555-9001
Home Phone: 999-555-7735			Employer's Address: 301 Valley Plaza	
Work Phone:			City: Fairview	State: OH	Zip: 43773
Spouse's Name:			Spouse's Employer:	
Emergency Contact: Ann Ferrone			Relationship: daughter	Phone #: 999-555-3237

FILL IN IF PATIENT IS A MINOR

Parent/Guardian's Name:	Sex:	Marital Status: ☐ S ☐ M ☐ D ☐ W	Birth Date:
Phone:	SS#:		
Address:	Employer:		Phone:
City: State: Zip:	Employer's Address:		
Student Status:	City: State: Zip:		

INSURANCE INFORMATION

Primary Insurance Company: Blue Cross/Blue Shield of Ohio	Secondary Insurance Company:
Subscriber's Name: Birth Date: Fran C. Ferrone 3/30/50	Subscriber's Name: Birth Date:
Plan: SS#: Traditional 332-75-9360	Plan:
Policy #: Group #: XRS332759360	Policy #: Group #:
Copayment/Deductible: Price Code: $500 deductible A	

OTHER INFORMATION

Reason for visit: cough	Allergy to Medication (list):
Name of referring physician:	If auto accident, list date and state in which it occurred:

I authorize treatment and agree to pay all fees and charges for the person named above. I agree to pay all charges shown by statements, promptly upon their presentation, unless credit arrangements are agreed upon in writing.

I authorize payment directly to POLARIS MEDICAL GROUP of insurance benefits otherwise payable to me. I hereby authorize the release of any medical information necessary in order to process a claim for payment in my behalf.

Fran C. Ferrone   6/21/10

(Patient's Signature/Parent or Guardian's Signature)   (Date)

I plan to make payment of my medical expenses as follows (check one or more):

X Insurance (as above)   X Cash/Check/Credit/Debit Card   ___ Medicare   ___ Medicaid   ___ Workers' Comp.

ENCOUNTER FORM

6/21/2010 9:00am	Dr. Robin Crebore
DATE TIME	PROVIDER
Fran C. Ferrone	FERROFR0
PATIENT NAME	CHART #

OFFICE VISITS - SYMPTOMATIC - NEW		
99201	OF--New Patient Minimal	
99202	OF--New Patient Low	X
99203	OF--New Patient Detailed	
99204	OF--New Patient Moderate	
99205	OF--New Patient High	

OFFICE VISITS - SYMPTOMATIC - ESTABLISHED		
99211	OF--Established Patient Minimal	
99212	OF--Established Patient Low	
99213	OF--Established Patient Detailed	
99214	OF--Established Patient Moderate	
99215	OF--Established Patient High	

PREVENTIVE VISITS - NEW		
99381	Under 1 Year	
99382	1 - 4 Years	
99383	5 - 11 Years	
99384	12 - 17 Years	
99385	18 - 39 Years	
99386	40 - 64 Years	
99387	65 Years & Up	

PREVENTIVE VISITS - ESTABLISHED		
99391	Under 1 Year	
99392	1 - 4 Years	
99393	5 - 11 Years	
99394	12 - 17 Years	
99395	18 - 39 Years	
99396	40 - 64 Years	
99397	65 Years & Up	

HOSPITAL/NURSING HOME VISITS		
99221	Initial hospital care, det.	
99222	Initial hospital care, comp.	
99223	Initial hospital care, high	
99281	ER Visit, min.	
99282	ER Visit, low	
99283	ER Visit, det.	
99284	ER Visit, moderate	
99285	ER Visit, high	
99307	Subseq. nursing facility care, pf.	

PROCEDURES		
10060	Incision/drainage, abcess	
20610	Aspiration, bursa	
29505	Splint, long leg	
29515	Splint, short leg	
36415	Routine venipuncture	
45330	Sigmoidoscopy, flex	
46600	Anoscopy, diagnostic	
71030	Chest x-ray, complete	
73610	Radiology, ankle, complete	
93000	Routine ECG	
93018	Cardiovascular stress test	
99070	Supplies and materials	

LABORATORY		
80050	General health panel	
81000	Urinalysis, complete	
82270	Blood, occult, feces screening	
82607	Vitamin B-12 test	
82948	Glucose, blood reagent	
85027	CBC, automated	
85651	Sedimentation rate test, manual	
86360	Absolute CD4/CD8 ratio	
86592	Syphilis test	
87070	Throat culture	
87088	Urine culture	
88150	Cytopathology, cervical or vaginal	

INJECTIONS		
90471	Immunization administration	
90472	Immunization administration, 2nd	
90658	Influenza injection, ages >3	
90702	DT immunization, ages <7	
90703	Tetanus immunization	
90707	MMR immunization	
90722	Therapeutic injection	
90723	DtaP - HepB - IPV	
90732	Pneumococcal immunization	

POLARIS MEDICAL GROUP

		NOTES
REFERRING PHYSICIAN	NPI	
AUTHORIZATION #		
DIAGNOSIS 490		
PAYMENT AMOUNT		

ENCOUNTER FORM

6/21/2010	9:30am	Dr. Michael Mahabir
DATE	TIME	PROVIDER

Jimmy R. Hellery	HELLEJI0
PATIENT NAME	CHART #

OFFICE VISITS - SYMPTOMATIC - NEW		
99201	OF--New Patient Minimal	
99202	OF--New Patient Low	
99203	OF--New Patient Detailed	
99204	OF--New Patient Moderate	
99205	OF--New Patient High	

OFFICE VISITS - SYMPTOMATIC - ESTABLISHED		
99211	OF--Established Patient Minimal	
99212	OF--Established Patient Low	X
99213	OF--Established Patient Detailed	
99214	OF--Established Patient Moderate	
99215	OF--Established Patient High	

PREVENTIVE VISITS - NEW		
99381	Under 1 Year	
99382	1 - 4 Years	
99383	5 - 11 Years	
99384	12 - 17 Years	
99385	18 - 39 Years	
99386	40 - 64 Years	
99387	65 Years & Up	

PREVENTIVE VISITS - ESTABLISHED		
99391	Under 1 Year	
99392	1 - 4 Years	
99393	5 - 11 Years	
99394	12 - 17 Years	
99395	18 - 39 Years	
99396	40 - 64 Years	
99397	65 Years & Up	

HOSPITAL/NURSING HOME VISITS		
99221	Initial hospital care, det.	
99222	Initial hospital care, comp.	
99223	Initial hospital care, high	
99281	ER Visit, min.	
99282	ER Visit, low	
99283	ER Visit, det.	
99284	ER Visit, moderate	
99285	ER Visit, high	
99307	Subseq. nursing facility care, pf.	

PROCEDURES		
10060	Incision/drainage, abcess	
20610	Aspiration, bursa	
29505	Splint, long leg	
29515	Splint, short leg	
36415	Routine venipuncture	
45330	Sigmoidoscopy, flex	
46600	Anoscopy, diagnostic	
71030	Chest x-ray, complete	
73610	Radiology, ankle, complete	
93000	Routine ECG	
93018	Cardiovascular stress test	
99070	Supplies and materials	

LABORATORY		
80050	General health panel	
81000	Urinalysis, complete	
82270	Blood, occult, feces screening	
82607	Vitamin B-12 test	
82948	Glucose, blood reagent	
85027	CBC, automated	
85651	Sedimentation rate test, manual	
86360	Absolute CD4/CD8 ratio	
86592	Syphilis test	
87070	Throat culture	X
87088	Urine culture	
88150	Cytopathology, cervical or vaginal	

INJECTIONS		
90471	Immunization administration	
90472	Immunization administration, 2nd	
90658	Influenza injection, ages >3	
90702	DT immunization, ages <7	
90703	Tetanus immunization	
90707	MMR immunization	
90722	Therapeutic injection	
90723	DtaP - HepB - IPV	
90732	Pneumococcal immunization	

POLARIS MEDICAL GROUP

REFERRING PHYSICIAN	NPI
AUTHORIZATION #	

NOTES

DIAGNOSIS
034.0

PAYMENT AMOUNT
$8.25 copay, check #1019

ENCOUNTER FORM

6/21/2010   **10:00am**
DATE   TIME

Floyd S. Deysenrothe
PATIENT NAME

Dr. Robin Crebore
PROVIDER

DEYSEFL0
CHART #

OFFICE VISITS - SYMPTOMATIC - NEW		
99201	OF--New Patient Minimal	
99202	OF--New Patient Low	
99203	OF--New Patient Detailed	
99204	OF--New Patient Moderate	
99205	OF--New Patient High	
OFFICE VISITS - SYMPTOMATIC - ESTABLISHED		
99211	OF--Established Patient Minimal	
99212	OF--Established Patient Low	
99213	OF--Established Patient Detailed	
99214	OF--Established Patient Moderate	
99215	OF--Established Patient High	
PREVENTIVE VISITS - NEW		
99381	Under 1 Year	
99382	1 - 4 Years	
99383	5 - 11 Years	
99384	12 - 17 Years	
99385	18 - 39 Years	
99386	40 - 64 Years	
99387	65 Years & Up	
PREVENTIVE VISITS - ESTABLISHED		
99391	Under 1 Year	
99392	1 - 4 Years	
99393	5 - 11 Years	
99394	12 - 17 Years	
99395	18 - 39 Years	
99396	40 - 64 Years	
99397	65 Years & Up	
HOSPITAL/NURSING HOME VISITS		
99221	Initial hospital care, det.	
99222	Initial hospital care, comp.	
99223	Initial hospital care, high	
99281	ER Visit, min.	
99282	ER Visit, low	
99283	ER Visit, det.	
99284	ER Visit, moderate	
99285	ER Visit, high	
99307	Subseq. nursing facility care, pf.	

PROCEDURES		
10060	Incision/drainage, abcess	
20610	Aspiration, bursa	
29505	Splint, long leg	
29515	Splint, short leg	
36415	Routine venipuncture	
45330	Sigmoidoscopy, flex	
46600	Anoscopy, diagnostic	
71030	Chest x-ray, complete	
73610	Radiology, ankle, complete	
93000	Routine ECG	
93018	Cardiovascular stress test	
99070	Supplies and materials	
LABORATORY		
80050	General health panel	
81000	Urinalysis, complete	
82270	Blood, occult, feces screening	
82607	Vitamin B-12 test	
82948	Glucose, blood reagent	
85027	CBC, automated	
85651	Sedimentation rate test, manual	
86360	Absolute CD4/CD8 ratio	
86592	Syphilis test	
87070	Throat culture	
87088	Urine culture	
88150	Cytopathology, cervical or vaginal	
INJECTIONS		
90471	Immunization administration	X
90472	Immunization administration, 2nd	
90658	Influenza injection, ages >3	
90702	DT immunization, ages <7	
90703	Tetanus immunization	X
90707	MMR immunization	
90722	Therapeutic injection	
90723	DtaP - HepB - IPV	
90732	Pneumococcal immunization	

POLARIS MEDICAL GROUP

NOTES

REFERRING PHYSICIAN

NPI

AUTHORIZATION #

DIAGNOSIS
v06.5

PAYMENT AMOUNT
$12.00 copay, check #1117

Blue Cross Blue Shield of Ohio
5000 First Street
Worthington, OH 43085

Polaris Medical Group
2100 Grace Avenue
Columbus, OH 43214

Practice ID: 04-5678901

Date Prepared: 6/21/10

EFT Number: 1238963

Patient's Name	Dates of Service From - Thru	POS	Proc	Qty	Charge Amount	Allowed Amount	Patient Resp.	Amt. Paid Provider
Brown, William	5/7/10 - 5/7/10	11	99213	1	$72.00	$72.00	$21.60	$50.40
Totals					$72.00	$72.00	$21.60	$50.40

* * * * * * * *EFT transmitted in the amount of $50.40* * * * * * * *

ENCOUNTER FORM

6/21/2010	4:15pm	Dr. Robin Crebore
DATE	TIME	PROVIDER

Elizabeth I. Wu	WUELIZA0
PATIENT NAME	CHART #

OFFICE VISITS - SYMPTOMATIC - NEW		
99201	OF--New Patient Minimal	
99202	OF--New Patient Low	
99203	OF--New Patient Detailed	
99204	OF--New Patient Moderate	
99205	OF--New Patient High	
OFFICE VISITS - SYMPTOMATIC - ESTABLISHED		
99211	OF--Established Patient Minimal	
99212	OF--Established Patient Low	X
99213	OF--Established Patient Detailed	
99214	OF--Established Patient Moderate	
99215	OF--Established Patient High	
PREVENTIVE VISITS - NEW		
99381	Under 1 Year	
99382	1 - 4 Years	
99383	5 - 11 Years	
99384	12 - 17 Years	
99385	18 - 39 Years	
99386	40 - 64 Years	
99387	65 Years & Up	
PREVENTIVE VISITS - ESTABLISHED		
99391	Under 1 Year	
99392	1 - 4 Years	
99393	5 - 11 Years	
99394	12 - 17 Years	
99395	18 - 39 Years	
99396	40 - 64 Years	
99397	65 Years & Up	
HOSPITAL/NURSING HOME VISITS		
99221	Initial hospital care, det.	
99222	Initial hospital care, comp.	
99223	Initial hospital care, high	
99281	ER Visit, min.	
99282	ER Visit, low	
99283	ER Visit, det.	
99284	ER Visit, moderate	
99285	ER Visit, high	
99307	Subseq. nursing facility care, pf.	

PROCEDURES		
10060	Incision/drainage, abcess	
20610	Aspiration, bursa	
29505	Splint, long leg	
29515	Splint, short leg	
36415	Routine venipuncture	
45330	Sigmoidoscopy, flex	
46600	Anoscopy, diagnostic	
71030	Chest x-ray, complete	
73610	Radiology, ankle, complete	
93000	Routine ECG	
93018	Cardiovascular stress test	
99070	Supplies and materials	
LABORATORY		
80050	General health panel	
81000	Urinalysis, complete	
82270	Blood, occult, feces screening	
82607	Vitamin B-12 test	
82948	Glucose, blood reagent	
85027	CBC, automated	
85651	Sedimentation rate test, manual	
86360	Absolute CD4/CD8 ratio	
86592	Syphilis test	
87070	Throat culture	
87088	Urine culture	
88150	Cytopathology, cervical or vaginal	
INJECTIONS		
90471	Immunization administration	
90472	Immunization administration, 2nd	
90658	Influenza injection, ages >3	
90702	DT immunization, ages <7	
90703	Tetanus immunization	
90707	MMR immunization	
90722	Therapeutic injection	
90723	DtaP - HepB - IPV	
90732	Pneumococcal immunization	

POLARIS MEDICAL GROUP		NOTES
REFERRING PHYSICIAN	NPI	
AUTHORIZATION #		
DIAGNOSIS 706.1		
PAYMENT AMOUNT $10.00 copay, check #1202		

Additional ICD Codes

Code	Description
v16.0	Family history of malignant neoplasm, GI tract
v24.2	Routine post-partum care—follow-up
794.31	Abnormal ECG
413.9	Angina pectoris
427.9	Cardiac dysrhythmia

ENCOUNTER FORM

6/22/2010	9:45am		Dr. Robin Crebore
DATE	TIME		PROVIDER

Flora K. Torres-Gil			TORREFL0
PATIENT NAME			CHART #

OFFICE VISITS - SYMPTOMATIC - NEW		
99201	OF--New Patient Minimal	
99202	OF--New Patient Low	
99203	OF--New Patient Detailed	
99204	OF--New Patient Moderate	
99205	OF--New Patient High	
OFFICE VISITS - SYMPTOMATIC - ESTABLISHED		
99211	OF--Established Patient Minimal	
99212	OF--Established Patient Low	
99213	OF--Established Patient Detailed	
99214	OF--Established Patient Moderate	
99215	OF--Established Patient High	
PREVENTIVE VISITS - NEW		
99381	Under 1 Year	
99382	1 - 4 Years	
99383	5 - 11 Years	
99384	12 - 17 Years	
99385	18 - 39 Years	
99386	40 - 64 Years	
99387	65 Years & Up	
PREVENTIVE VISITS - ESTABLISHED		
99391	Under 1 Year	
99392	1 - 4 Years	
99393	5 - 11 Years	
99394	12 - 17 Years	
99395	18 - 39 Years	
99396	40 - 64 Years	
99397	65 Years & Up	
HOSPITAL/NURSING HOME VISITS		
99221	Initial hospital care, det.	
99222	Initial hospital care, comp.	
99223	Initial hospital care, high	
99281	ER Visit, min.	
99282	ER Visit, low	
99283	ER Visit, det.	
99284	ER Visit, moderate	
99285	ER Visit, high	
99307	Subseq. nursing facility care, pf.	

PROCEDURES		
10060	Incision/drainage, abcess	
20610	Aspiration, bursa	X
29505	Splint, long leg	
29515	Splint, short leg	
36415	Routine venipuncture	
45330	Sigmoidoscopy, flex	
46600	Anoscopy, diagnostic	
71030	Chest x-ray, complete	
73610	Radiology, ankle, complete	
93000	Routine ECG	
93018	Cardiovascular stress test	
99070	Supplies and materials	
LABORATORY		
80050	General health panel	
81000	Urinalysis, complete	
82270	Blood, occult, feces screening	
82607	Vitamin B-12 test	
82948	Glucose, blood reagent	
85027	CBC, automated	
85651	Sedimentation rate test, manual	
86360	Absolute CD4/CD8 ratio	
86592	Syphilis test	
87070	Throat culture	
87088	Urine culture	
88150	Cytopathology, cervical or vaginal	
INJECTIONS		
90471	Immunization administration	
90472	Immunization administration, 2nd	
90658	Influenza injection, ages >3	
90702	DT immunization, ages <7	
90703	Tetanus immunization	
90707	MMR immunization	
90722	Therapeutic injection	
90723	DtaP - HepB - IPV	
90732	Pneumococcal immunization	

POLARIS MEDICAL GROUP

REFERRING PHYSICIAN	NPI

AUTHORIZATION #

DIAGNOSIS
727.3

PAYMENT AMOUNT
$5.00 copay, check #1309

NOTES

Information on Ohio Maxcare PPO, 6/22/2010

Ohio Maxcare PPO

4001 Bridgeway Center

Columbus, OH 43214

Phone: 800-555-0060

Fax: 999-555-8814

Representative: Sharon Lucas

Practice ID: 01-765432

Plan Name/Type: Maxcare

Billing Method: Electronic

EDI Receiver: NDCO

EDI Payor Number: 0123

EDI Sub ID: 456

NDC Record Code: 07

Codes:

Payment: PAYMAX

Adjustment: ADJMAX

Withhold: WITMAX

Deductible: DEDMAX

Take Back: TBKMAX

Allowed Amounts: Refer to SD 48

PINs: Leave blank.

POLARIS MEDICAL GROUP
Discounted Fee Schedule: Ohio Maxcare PPO

OFFICE VISITS - SYMPTOMATIC

NEW
99201	OF-New Patient Minimal	56
99202	OF-New Patient Low	75
99203	OF-New Patient Detailed	103
99204	OF-New Patient Moderate	150
99205	OF-New Patient High	194

ESTABLISHED
99211	OF-Est. Patient Minimal	30
99212	OF-Est. Patient Low	46
99213	OF-Est. Patient Detailed	62
99214	OF-Est. Patient Moderate	91
99215	OF-Est. Patient High	140

PREVENTIVE VISITS

NEW
99381	Under 1 Year	140
99382	1 - 4 Years	146
99383	5 - 11 Years	143
99384	12 - 17 Years	178
99385	18 - 39 Years	166
99386	40 - 64 Years	180
99387	65 Years & Up	200

ESTABLISHED
99391	Under 1 Year	111
99392	1 - 4 Years	124
99393	5 - 11 Years	130
99394	12 - 17 Years	149
99395	18 - 39 Years	137
99396	40 - 64 Years	149
99397	65 Years & Up	120

HOSPITAL/NURSING HOME VISITS
99221	Initial hospital care, det.	160
99222	Initial hospital care, comp.	177
99223	Initial hospital care, high	218
99281	ER visit, min.	87
99282	ER visit, low	109
99283	ER visit, det.	131
99284	ER visit, moderate	153
99285	ER visit, high	175
99307	Subseq. nursing facility care, pf.	54

PROCEDURES
10060	Incision/drainage, abcess	98
20610	Aspiration, bursa	91
29505	Splint, long leg	110
29515	Splint, short leg	94
36415	Routine venipuncture	17
45330	Sigmoidoscopy, flex	226
46600	Anoscopy, collection	72
71030	Chest x-ray, complete	128
73610	Radiology, ankle, complete	94
93000	Routine ECG	70
93018	Cardiovascular stress test	162
99070	Supplies and materials	-----

LABORATORY
80050	General health panel	120
81000	Urinalysis, complete	17
82270	Blood, occult, feces screening	15
82607	Vitamin B-12 test	72
82948	Glucose, blood reagent	15
85027	CBC, automated	27
85651	Sedimentation rate test, manual	20
86360	Absolute CD4/CD8 ratio	195
86592	Syphilis test	20
87070	Throat culture	38
87088	Urine culture	34
88150	Cytopathology, cervical or vaginal	29

INJECTIONS
90471	Immunization administration	14
90472	Immunization administration, 2nd	8
90658	Influenza injection, ages >3	23
90702	DT immunization, ages <7	27
90703	Tetanus immunization	24
90707	MMR immunization	75
90722	Therapeutic injection	20
90723	DtaP - HepB - IPV	67
90732	Pneumococcal immunization	32

ENCOUNTER FORM

6/22/2010 10:45am	Dr. Robin Crebore
DATE TIME	PROVIDER
Diana E. O'Keefe	OKEEFDI0
PATIENT NAME	CHART #

OFFICE VISITS - SYMPTOMATIC - NEW		
99201	OF--New Patient Minimal	
99202	OF--New Patient Low	
99203	OF--New Patient Detailed	
99204	OF--New Patient Moderate	
99205	OF--New Patient High	
OFFICE VISITS - SYMPTOMATIC - ESTABLISHED		
99211	OF--Established Patient Minimal	X
99212	OF--Established Patient Low	
99213	OF--Established Patient Detailed	
99214	OF--Established Patient Moderate	
99215	OF--Established Patient High	
PREVENTIVE VISITS - NEW		
99381	Under 1 Year	
99382	1 - 4 Years	
99383	5 - 11 Years	
99384	12 - 17 Years	
99385	18 - 39 Years	
99386	40 - 64 Years	
99387	65 Years & Up	
PREVENTIVE VISITS - ESTABLISHED		
99391	Under 1 Year	
99392	1 - 4 Years	
99393	5 - 11 Years	
99394	12 - 17 Years	
99395	18 - 39 Years	
99396	40 - 64 Years	
99397	65 Years & Up	
HOSPITAL/NURSING HOME VISITS		
99221	Initial hospital care, det.	
99222	Initial hospital care, comp.	
99223	Initial hospital care, high	
99281	ER Visit, min.	
99282	ER Visit, low	
99283	ER Visit, det.	
99284	ER Visit, moderate	
99285	ER Visit, high	
99307	Subseq. nursing facility care, pf.	

PROCEDURES		
10060	Incision/drainage, abcess	
20610	Aspiration, bursa	
29505	Splint, long leg	
29515	Splint, short leg	
36415	Routine venipuncture	
45330	Sigmoidoscopy, flex	
46600	Anoscopy, diagnostic	
71030	Chest x-ray, complete	
73610	Radiology, ankle, complete	
93000	Routine ECG	
93018	Cardiovascular stress test	
99070	Supplies and materials	
LABORATORY		
80050	General health panel	
81000	Urinalysis, complete	
82270	Blood, occult, feces screening	
82607	Vitamin B-12 test	
82948	Glucose, blood reagent	
85027	CBC, automated	
85651	Sedimentation rate test, manual	X
86360	Absolute CD4/CD8 ratio	
86592	Syphilis test	
87070	Throat culture	
87088	Urine culture	
88150	Cytopathology, cervical or vaginal	
INJECTIONS		
90471	Immunization administration	
90472	Immunization administration, 2nd	
90658	Influenza injection, ages >3	
90702	DT immunization, ages <7	
90703	Tetanus immunization	
90707	MMR immunization	
90722	Therapeutic injection	
90723	DtaP - HepB - IPV	
90732	Pneumococcal immunization	

POLARIS MEDICAL GROUP

		NOTES
REFERRING PHYSICIAN	NPI	
AUTHORIZATION #		
DIAGNOSIS		
714.0		
PAYMENT AMOUNT		

ENCOUNTER FORM

6/23/2010 DATE	**9:00am** TIME	**Dr. Robin Crebore** PROVIDER
Felidia E. Jonas PATIENT NAME		**JONASFE0** CHART #

OFFICE VISITS - SYMPTOMATIC - NEW		
99201	OF--New Patient Minimal	
99202	OF--New Patient Low	
99203	OF--New Patient Detailed	
99204	OF--New Patient Moderate	
99205	OF--New Patient High	
OFFICE VISITS - SYMPTOMATIC - ESTABLISHED		
99211	OF--Established Patient Minimal	X
99212	OF--Established Patient Low	
99213	OF--Established Patient Detailed	
99214	OF--Established Patient Moderate	
99215	OF--Established Patient High	
PREVENTIVE VISITS - NEW		
99381	Under 1 Year	
99382	1 - 4 Years	
99383	5 - 11 Years	
99384	12 - 17 Years	
99385	18 - 39 Years	
99386	40 - 64 Years	
99387	65 Years & Up	
PREVENTIVE VISITS - ESTABLISHED		
99391	Under 1 Year	
99392	1 - 4 Years	
99393	5 - 11 Years	
99394	12 - 17 Years	
99395	18 - 39 Years	
99396	40 - 64 Years	
99397	65 Years & Up	
HOSPITAL/NURSING HOME VISITS		
99221	Initial hospital care, det.	
99222	Initial hospital care, comp.	
99223	Initial hospital care, high	
99281	ER Visit, min.	
99282	ER Visit, low	
99283	ER Visit, det.	
99284	ER Visit, moderate	
99285	ER Visit, high	
99307	Subseq. nursing facility care, pf.	

PROCEDURES		
10060	Incision/drainage, abcess	
20610	Aspiration, bursa	
29505	Splint, long leg	
29515	Splint, short leg	
36415	Routine venipuncture	
45330	Sigmoidoscopy, flex	
46600	Anoscopy, diagnostic	
71030	Chest x-ray, complete	
73610	Radiology, ankle, complete	
93000	Routine ECG	
93018	Cardiovascular stress test	
99070	Supplies and materials	
LABORATORY		
80050	General health panel	
81000	Urinalysis, complete	
82270	Blood, occult, feces screening	
82607	Vitamin B-12 test	
82948	Glucose, blood reagent	
85027	CBC, automated	
85651	Sedimentation rate test, manual	
86360	Absolute CD4/CD8 ratio	
86592	Syphilis test	
87070	Throat culture	
87088	Urine culture	
88150	Cytopathology, cervical or vaginal	
INJECTIONS		
90471	Immunization administration	
90472	Immunization administration, 2nd	
90658	Influenza injection, ages >3	
90702	DT immunization, ages <7	
90703	Tetanus immunization	
90707	MMR immunization	
90722	Therapeutic injection	
90723	DtaP - HepB - IPV	
90732	Pneumococcal immunization	

POLARIS MEDICAL GROUP

		NOTES
REFERRING PHYSICIAN	NPI	
AUTHORIZATION #		
DIAGNOSIS 684		
PAYMENT AMOUNT $15.00 copay, check #2349		

ENCOUNTER FORM

6/23/2010	10:00am	Dr. Robin Crebore
DATE	TIME	PROVIDER

Cynthia I. Cashell	CASHECY0
PATIENT NAME	CHART #

OFFICE VISITS - SYMPTOMATIC - NEW		
99201	OF--New Patient Minimal	
99202	OF--New Patient Low	
99203	OF--New Patient Detailed	
99204	OF--New Patient Moderate	
99205	OF--New Patient High	
OFFICE VISITS - SYMPTOMATIC - ESTABLISHED		
99211	OF--Established Patient Minimal	
99212	OF--Established Patient Low	
99213	OF--Established Patient Detailed	
99214	OF--Established Patient Moderate	X
99215	OF--Established Patient High	
PREVENTIVE VISITS - NEW		
99381	Under 1 Year	
99382	1 - 4 Years	
99383	5 - 11 Years	
99384	12 - 17 Years	
99385	18 - 39 Years	
99386	40 - 64 Years	
99387	65 Years & Up	
PREVENTIVE VISITS - ESTABLISHED		
99391	Under 1 Year	
99392	1 - 4 Years	
99393	5 - 11 Years	
99394	12 - 17 Years	
99395	18 - 39 Years	
99396	40 - 64 Years	
99397	65 Years & Up	
HOSPITAL/NURSING HOME VISITS		
99221	Initial hospital care, det.	
99222	Initial hospital care, comp.	
99223	Initial hospital care, high	
99281	ER Visit, min.	
99282	ER Visit, low	
99283	ER Visit, det.	
99284	ER Visit, moderate	
99285	ER Visit, high	
99307	Subseq. nursing facility care, pf.	

PROCEDURES		
10060	Incision/drainage, abcess	
20610	Aspiration, bursa	
29505	Splint, long leg	
29515	Splint, short leg	
36415	Routine venipuncture	
45330	Sigmoidoscopy, flex	
46600	Anoscopy, diagnostic	
71030	Chest x-ray, complete	
73610	Radiology, ankle, complete	
93000	Routine ECG	
93018	Cardiovascular stress test	
99070	Supplies and materials	X
LABORATORY		
80050	General health panel	
81000	Urinalysis, complete	
82270	Blood, occult, feces screening	
82607	Vitamin B-12 test	
82948	Glucose, blood reagent	
85027	CBC, automated	
85651	Sedimentation rate test, manual	
86360	Absolute CD4/CD8 ratio	
86592	Syphilis test	
87070	Throat culture	
87088	Urine culture	
88150	Cytopathology, cervical or vaginal	
INJECTIONS		
90471	Immunization administration	
90472	Immunization administration, 2nd	
90658	Influenza injection, ages >3	
90702	DT immunization, ages <7	
90703	Tetanus immunization	
90707	MMR immunization	
90722	Therapeutic injection	
90723	DtaP - HepB - IPV	
90732	Pneumococcal immunization	

POLARIS MEDICAL GROUP

REFERRING PHYSICIAN	NPI	NOTES
		99070 supplies and materials $20.00
AUTHORIZATION #		
DIAGNOSIS 696.1		
PAYMENT AMOUNT $125, check #102		

PATIENT INFORMATION FORM

THIS SECTION REFERS TO PATIENT ONLY

Name: Chantalle E. Usdan	Sex: F	Marital Status: ☒ S ☐ M ☐ D ☐ W	Birth Date: 2/23/54

Address: 28 Fairview Blvd.	SS#: 234-60-8721		

City: Columbus	State: OH	Zip: 43214	Employer: Argene Interiors (full-time)	Phone:

Home Phone: 999-555-4555	Employer's Address: 1760 Watertown Avenue		

Work Phone: 999-555-6978	City: Jackson	State: OH	Zip: 45640

Spouse's Name:	Spouse's Employer:

Emergency Contact: Laraine Modell	Relationship: sister	Phone #: 999-555-9910

FILL IN IF PATIENT IS A MINOR

Parent/Guardian's Name:	Sex:	Marital Status: ☐ S ☐ M ☐ D ☐ W	Birth Date:

Phone:	SS#:		

Address:	Employer:	Phone:

City:	State:	Zip:	Employer's Address:		

Student Status:	City:	State:	Zip:

INSURANCE INFORMATION

Primary Insurance Company: Cigna Healthplan	Secondary Insurance Company:

Subscriber's Name: Chantalle E. Usdan	Birth Date: 2/23/54	Subscriber's Name:	Birth Date:

Plan: HMO	SS#: 234-60-8721	Plan:

Policy #: 723-C48	Group #: AAA66668	Policy #:	Group #:

Copayment/Deductible: $18 copay	Price Code: A	

OTHER INFORMATION

Reason for visit: flexible sigmoidoscopy	Allergy to Medication (list):

Name of referring physician: Dr. Rachel P. Innanni	If auto accident, list date and state in which it occurred:

I authorize treatment and agree to pay all fees and charges for the person named above. I agree to pay all charges shown by statements, promptly upon their presentation, unless credit arrangements are agreed upon in writing.

I authorize payment directly to POLARIS MEDICAL GROUP of insurance benefits otherwise payable to me. I hereby authorize the release of any medical information necessary in order to process a claim for payment in my behalf.

Chantalle E. Usdan	6/23/10
(Patient's Signature/Parent or Guardian's Signature)	(Date)

I plan to make payment of my medical expenses as follows (check one or more):

__X__ Insurance (as above)   __X__ Cash/Check/Credit/Debit Card   _____ Medicare   _____ Medicaid   _____ Workers' Comp.

ENCOUNTER FORM

6/23/2010   10:00am
DATE   TIME

Dr. Michael Mahabir
PROVIDER

Chantalle E. Usdan
PATIENT NAME

USDANCH0
CHART #

OFFICE VISITS - SYMPTOMATIC - NEW		
99201	OF--New Patient Minimal	
99202	OF--New Patient Low	
99203	OF--New Patient Detailed	
99204	OF--New Patient Moderate	
99205	OF--New Patient High	
OFFICE VISITS - SYMPTOMATIC - ESTABLISHED		
99211	OF--Established Patient Minimal	
99212	OF--Established Patient Low	
99213	OF--Established Patient Detailed	
99214	OF--Established Patient Moderate	
99215	OF--Established Patient High	
PREVENTIVE VISITS - NEW		
99381	Under 1 Year	
99382	1 - 4 Years	
99383	5 - 11 Years	
99384	12 - 17 Years	
99385	18 - 39 Years	
99386	40 - 64 Years	
99387	65 Years & Up	
PREVENTIVE VISITS - ESTABLISHED		
99391	Under 1 Year	
99392	1 - 4 Years	
99393	5 - 11 Years	
99394	12 - 17 Years	
99395	18 - 39 Years	
99396	40 - 64 Years	
99397	65 Years & Up	
HOSPITAL/NURSING HOME VISITS		
99221	Initial hospital care, det.	
99222	Initial hospital care, comp.	
99223	Initial hospital care, high	
99281	ER Visit, min.	
99282	ER Visit, low	
99283	ER Visit, det.	
99284	ER Visit, moderate	
99285	ER Visit, high	
99307	Subseq. nursing facility care, pf.	

PROCEDURES		
10060	Incision/drainage, abcess	
20610	Aspiration, bursa	
29505	Splint, long leg	
29515	Splint, short leg	
36415	Routine venipuncture	
45330	Sigmoidoscopy, flex	X
46600	Anoscopy, diagnostic	
71030	Chest x-ray, complete	
73610	Radiology, ankle, complete	
93000	Routine ECG	
93018	Cardiovascular stress test	
99070	Supplies and materials	
LABORATORY		
80050	General health panel	
81000	Urinalysis, complete	
82270	Blood, occult, feces screening	
82607	Vitamin B-12 test	
82948	Glucose, blood reagent	
85027	CBC, automated	
85651	Sedimentation rate test, manual	
86360	Absolute CD4/CD8 ratio	
86592	Syphilis test	
87070	Throat culture	
87088	Urine culture	
88150	Cytopathology, cervical or vaginal	
INJECTIONS		
90471	Immunization administration	
90472	Immunization administration, 2nd	
90658	Influenza injection, ages >3	
90702	DT immunization, ages <7	
90703	Tetanus immunization	
90707	MMR immunization	
90722	Therapeutic injection	
90723	DtaP - HepB - IPV	
90732	Pneumococcal immunization	

POLARIS MEDICAL GROUP

REFERRING PHYSICIAN	NPI	NOTES
Dr. Rachel Innanni		

AUTHORIZATION #

DIAGNOSIS

PAYMENT AMOUNT
$18.00 copay, check #409

ENCOUNTER FORM

6/23/2010 12:00pm	Dr. Michael Mahabir
DATE TIME	PROVIDER
Rachel D. Atchely	ATCHERA0
PATIENT NAME	CHART #

OFFICE VISITS - SYMPTOMATIC - NEW

Code	Description	
99201	OF--New Patient Minimal	
99202	OF--New Patient Low	
99203	OF--New Patient Detailed	
99204	OF--New Patient Moderate	
99205	OF--New Patient High	

OFFICE VISITS - SYMPTOMATIC - ESTABLISHED

Code	Description	
99211	OF--Established Patient Minimal	
99212	OF--Established Patient Low	
99213	OF--Established Patient Detailed	
99214	OF--Established Patient Moderate	
99215	OF--Established Patient High	

PREVENTIVE VISITS - NEW

Code	Description	
99381	Under 1 Year	
99382	1 - 4 Years	
99383	5 - 11 Years	
99384	12 - 17 Years	
99385	18 - 39 Years	
99386	40 - 64 Years	
99387	65 Years & Up	

PREVENTIVE VISITS - ESTABLISHED

Code	Description	
99391	Under 1 Year	
99392	1 - 4 Years	
99393	5 - 11 Years	
99394	12 - 17 Years	
99395	18 - 39 Years	
99396	40 - 64 Years	
99397	65 Years & Up	

HOSPITAL/NURSING HOME VISITS

Code	Description	
99221	Initial hospital care, det.	
99222	Initial hospital care, comp.	
99223	Initial hospital care, high	
99281	ER Visit, min.	
99282	ER Visit, low	
99283	ER Visit, det.	
99284	ER Visit, moderate	
99285	ER Visit, high	
99307	Subseq. nursing facility care, pf.	X

PROCEDURES

Code	Description	
10060	Incision/drainage, abcess	
20610	Aspiration, bursa	
29505	Splint, long leg	
29515	Splint, short leg	
36415	Routine venipuncture	
45330	Sigmoidoscopy, flex	
46600	Anoscopy, diagnostic	
71030	Chest x-ray, complete	
73610	Radiology, ankle, complete	
93000	Routine ECG	
93018	Cardiovascular stress test	
99070	Supplies and materials	

LABORATORY

Code	Description	
80050	General health panel	
81000	Urinalysis, complete	
82270	Blood, occult, feces screening	
82607	Vitamin B-12 test	
82948	Glucose, blood reagent	
85027	CBC, automated	
85651	Sedimentation rate test, manual	
86360	Absolute CD4/CD8 ratio	
86592	Syphilis test	
87070	Throat culture	
87088	Urine culture	
88150	Cytopathology, cervical or vaginal	

INJECTIONS

Code	Description	
90471	Immunization administration	
90472	Immunization administration, 2nd	
90658	Influenza injection, ages >3	
90702	DT immunization, ages <7	
90703	Tetanus immunization	
90707	MMR immunization	
90722	Therapeutic injection	
90723	DtaP - HepB - IPV	
90732	Pneumococcal immunization	

POLARIS MEDICAL GROUP

REFERRING PHYSICIAN	NPI	NOTES
AUTHORIZATION #		
DIAGNOSIS 682.7		
PAYMENT AMOUNT $5.00 copay, check #1078		

ENCOUNTER FORM

6/23/2010	2:15pm	Dr. Michael Mahabir
DATE	TIME	PROVIDER

Mae J. Deysenrothe	DEYSEMA0
PATIENT NAME	CHART #

OFFICE VISITS - SYMPTOMATIC - NEW		
99201	OF--New Patient Minimal	
99202	OF--New Patient Low	
99203	OF--New Patient Detailed	
99204	OF--New Patient Moderate	
99205	OF--New Patient High	
OFFICE VISITS - SYMPTOMATIC - ESTABLISHED		
99211	OF--Established Patient Minimal	
99212	OF--Established Patient Low	
99213	OF--Established Patient Detailed	
99214	OF--Established Patient Moderate	
99215	OF--Established Patient High	
PREVENTIVE VISITS - NEW		
99381	Under 1 Year	
99382	1 - 4 Years	
99383	5 - 11 Years	
99384	12 - 17 Years	
99385	18 - 39 Years	
99386	40 - 64 Years	
99387	65 Years & Up	
PREVENTIVE VISITS - ESTABLISHED		
99391	Under 1 Year	
99392	1 - 4 Years	
99393	5 - 11 Years	
99394	12 - 17 Years	
99395	18 - 39 Years	X
99396	40 - 64 Years	
99397	65 Years & Up	
HOSPITAL/NURSING HOME VISITS		
99221	Initial hospital care, det.	
99222	Initial hospital care, comp.	
99223	Initial hospital care, high	
99281	ER Visit, min.	
99282	ER Visit, low	
99283	ER Visit, det.	
99284	ER Visit, moderate	
99285	ER Visit, high	
99307	Subseq. nursing facility care, pf.	

PROCEDURES		
10060	Incision/drainage, abcess	
20610	Aspiration, bursa	
29505	Splint, long leg	
29515	Splint, short leg	
36415	Routine venipuncture	X
45330	Sigmoidoscopy, flex	
46600	Anoscopy, diagnostic	
71030	Chest x-ray, complete	
73610	Radiology, ankle, complete	
93000	Routine ECG	X
93018	Cardiovascular stress test	
99070	Supplies and materials	
LABORATORY		
80050	General health panel	X
81000	Urinalysis, complete	X
82270	Blood, occult, feces screening	
82607	Vitamin B-12 test	
82948	Glucose, blood reagent	
85027	CBC, automated	
85651	Sedimentation rate test, manual	
86360	Absolute CD4/CD8 ratio	
86592	Syphilis test	
87070	Throat culture	
87088	Urine culture	
88150	Cytopathology, cervical or vaginal	X
INJECTIONS		
90471	Immunization administration	
90472	Immunization administration, 2nd	
90658	Influenza injection, ages >3	
90702	DT immunization, ages <7	
90703	Tetanus immunization	
90707	MMR immunization	
90722	Therapeutic injection	
90723	DtaP - HepB - IPV	
90732	Pneumococcal immunization	

POLARIS MEDICAL GROUP

REFERRING PHYSICIAN	NPI

AUTHORIZATION #

DIAGNOSIS
v70.0

PAYMENT AMOUNT
$12.00 copay, check #2043

NOTES

ENCOUNTER FORM

6/23/2010 4:30pm	Dr. Michael Mahabir
DATE TIME	PROVIDER
Ann R. LeConey	LECONAN0
PATIENT NAME	CHART #

OFFICE VISITS - SYMPTOMATIC - NEW		
99201	OF--New Patient Minimal	
99202	OF--New Patient Low	
99203	OF--New Patient Detailed	
99204	OF--New Patient Moderate	
99205	OF--New Patient High	

OFFICE VISITS - SYMPTOMATIC - ESTABLISHED		
99211	OF--Established Patient Minimal	
99212	OF--Established Patient Low	X
99213	OF--Established Patient Detailed	
99214	OF--Established Patient Moderate	
99215	OF--Established Patient High	

PREVENTIVE VISITS - NEW		
99381	Under 1 Year	
99382	1 - 4 Years	
99383	5 - 11 Years	
99384	12 - 17 Years	
99385	18 - 39 Years	
99386	40 - 64 Years	
99387	65 Years & Up	

PREVENTIVE VISITS - ESTABLISHED		
99391	Under 1 Year	
99392	1 - 4 Years	
99393	5 - 11 Years	
99394	12 - 17 Years	
99395	18 - 39 Years	
99396	40 - 64 Years	
99397	65 Years & Up	

HOSPITAL/NURSING HOME VISITS		
99221	Initial hospital care, det.	
99222	Initial hospital care, comp.	
99223	Initial hospital care, high	
99281	ER Visit, min.	
99282	ER Visit, low	
99283	ER Visit, det.	
99284	ER Visit, moderate	
99285	ER Visit, high	
99307	Subseq. nursing facility care, pf.	

PROCEDURES		
10060	Incision/drainage, abcess	
20610	Aspiration, bursa	
29505	Splint, long leg	
29515	Splint, short leg	
36415	Routine venipuncture	
45330	Sigmoidoscopy, flex	
46600	Anoscopy, diagnostic	
71030	Chest x-ray, complete	
73610	Radiology, ankle, complete	
93000	Routine ECG	
93018	Cardiovascular stress test	
99070	Supplies and materials	

LABORATORY		
80050	General health panel	
81000	Urinalysis, complete	
82270	Blood, occult, feces screening	
82607	Vitamin B-12 test	
82948	Glucose, blood reagent	
85027	CBC, automated	
85651	Sedimentation rate test, manual	
86360	Absolute CD4/CD8 ratio	
86592	Syphilis test	
87070	Throat culture	
87088	Urine culture	
88150	Cytopathology, cervical or vaginal	

INJECTIONS		
90471	Immunization administration	
90472	Immunization administration, 2nd	
90658	Influenza injection, ages >3	
90702	DT immunization, ages <7	
90703	Tetanus immunization	
90707	MMR immunization	
90722	Therapeutic injection	
90723	DtaP - HepB - IPV	
90732	Pneumococcal immunization	

POLARIS MEDICAL GROUP		NOTES
REFERRING PHYSICIAN	NPI	
AUTHORIZATION #		
DIAGNOSIS 701.9		
PAYMENT AMOUNT $15.00 copay, check #1834		

PATIENT INFORMATION FORM

THIS SECTION REFERS TO PATIENT ONLY

Name: Hanna Z. Wong	Sex: F	Marital Status: ☐ S ☐ M ☐ D ☒ W	Birth Date: 11/5/37

Address: 22-B 22nd Avenue	SS#: 015-98-2139

City: Highland	State: OH	Zip: 45132	Employer: retired	Phone:

Home Phone: 999-555-1122	Employer's Address:

Work Phone:	City:	State:	Zip:

Spouse's Name:	Spouse's Employer:

Emergency Contact: John Wong	Relationship: son	Phone #: 999-555-0364

FILL IN IF PATIENT IS A MINOR

Parent/Guardian's Name:	Sex:	Marital Status: ☐ S ☐ M ☐ D ☐ W	Birth Date:

Phone:	SS#:

Address:	Employer:	Phone:

City:	State:	Zip:	Employer's Address:	

Student Status:	City:	State:	Zip:

INSURANCE INFORMATION

Primary Insurance Company: Nationwide Medicare HMO	Secondary Insurance Company:

Subscriber's Name: Hanna Wong	Birth Date: 11/5/37	Subscriber's Name:	Birth Date:

Plan: HMO	SS#: 015-98-2139	Plan:

Policy #: 015-98-2139A	Group #:	Policy #:	Group #:

Copayment/Deductible: $5 copay	Price Code: A	

OTHER INFORMATION

Reason for visit: chest pain when lifting	Allergy to Medication (list):

Name of referring physician:	If auto accident, list date and state in which it occurred:

I authorize treatment and agree to pay all fees and charges for the person named above. I agree to pay all charges shown by statements, promptly upon their presentation, unless credit arrangements are agreed upon in writing.

I authorize payment directly to POLARIS MEDICAL GROUP of insurance benefits otherwise payable to me. I hereby authorize the release of any medical information necessary in order to process a claim for payment in my behalf.

Hanna Wong	6/24/10
(Patient's Signature/Parent or Guardian's Signature)	(Date)

I plan to make payment of my medical expenses as follows (check one or more):

_____ Insurance (as above)   _X_ Cash/Check/Credit/Debit Card   _X_ Medicare   _____ Medicaid   _____ Workers' Comp.

ENCOUNTER FORM

6/24/2010 **10:00am**	**Dr. Michael Mahabir**
DATE TIME	PROVIDER
Hanna Z. Wong	**WONGHAN0**
PATIENT NAME	CHART #

OFFICE VISITS - SYMPTOMATIC - NEW		
99201	OF--New Patient Minimal	
99202	OF--New Patient Low	
99203	OF--New Patient Detailed	
99204	OF--New Patient Moderate	
99205	OF--New Patient High	X
OFFICE VISITS - SYMPTOMATIC - ESTABLISHED		
99211	OF--Established Patient Minimal	
99212	OF--Established Patient Low	
99213	OF--Established Patient Detailed	
99214	OF--Established Patient Moderate	
99215	OF--Established Patient High	
PREVENTIVE VISITS - NEW		
99381	Under 1 Year	
99382	1 - 4 Years	
99383	5 - 11 Years	
99384	12 - 17 Years	
99385	18 - 39 Years	
99386	40 - 64 Years	
99387	65 Years & Up	
PREVENTIVE VISITS - ESTABLISHED		
99391	Under 1 Year	
99392	1 - 4 Years	
99393	5 - 11 Years	
99394	12 - 17 Years	
99395	18 - 39 Years	
99396	40 - 64 Years	
99397	65 Years & Up	
HOSPITAL/NURSING HOME VISITS		
99221	Initial hospital care, det.	
99222	Initial hospital care, comp.	
99223	Initial hospital care, high	
99281	ER Visit, min.	
99282	ER Visit, low	
99283	ER Visit, det.	
99284	ER Visit, moderate	
99285	ER Visit, high	
99307	Subseq. nursing facility care, pf.	

PROCEDURES		
10060	Incision/drainage, abcess	
20610	Aspiration, bursa	
29505	Splint, long leg	
29515	Splint, short leg	
36415	Routine venipuncture	
45330	Sigmoidoscopy, flex	
46600	Anoscopy, diagnostic	
71030	Chest x-ray, complete	
73610	Radiology, ankle, complete	
93000	Routine ECG	X
93018	Cardiovascular stress test	
99070	Supplies and materials	
LABORATORY		
80050	General health panel	
81000	Urinalysis, complete	
82270	Blood, occult, feces screening	
82607	Vitamin B-12 test	
82948	Glucose, blood reagent	
85027	CBC, automated	
85651	Sedimentation rate test, manual	
86360	Absolute CD4/CD8 ratio	
86592	Syphilis test	
87070	Throat culture	
87088	Urine culture	
88150	Cytopathology, cervical or vaginal	
INJECTIONS		
90471	Immunization administration	
90472	Immunization administration, 2nd	
90658	Influenza injection, ages >3	
90702	DT immunization, ages <7	
90703	Tetanus immunization	
90707	MMR immunization	
90722	Therapeutic injection	
90723	DtaP - HepB - IPV	
90732	Pneumococcal immunization	

POLARIS MEDICAL GROUP

			NOTES
REFERRING PHYSICIAN		NPI	
AUTHORIZATION #			
DIAGNOSIS			
786.50			
PAYMENT AMOUNT			
$5.00 copay, check #840			

Electronic Claim Audit/Edit Report

Polaris Medical Group
2100 Grace Avenue
Columbus, OH 43214

Transmission Number: 6084998

Insurance Carrier: Medicare

Patient's Name	Dates of Service From - Thru	POS	Proc	Qty	Status
Connolly, Daniel	6/3/10 - 6/3/10	11	99397	1	Rejected**A
Connolly, Daniel	6/3/10 - 6/3/10	11	80050	1	Rejected**A

** see reason for rejection below

**A Procedure not covered

Additional CPT Codes

Code	Description	POS	Charge A
74240**	X-ray exam, upper GI tract	11	$88.00
74290**	Contrast X-ray, gallbladder	11	$130.00

** Require modifier -26, interpretation only

Insurance Company Allowed Amounts:

Insurance Name	Code 74240	Code 74290
Aetna Health Plans	$ 74.00	$108.00
BCBS of Ohio - Workers' Comp.	88.00	130.00
Blue Cross/Blue Shield of Ohio	88.00	130.00
CIGNA Healthplan	74.00	108.00
Columbus Medical Care	74.00	108.00
Nationwide Medicare (HMO)	36.00	68.00
Nationwide Medicare (Trad)	36.00	68.00
Ohio Depart. of Human Services	36.00	68.00
Ohio Insurance Company	88.00	130.00
Ohio Maxcare PPO	74.00	108.00
Standard Health Care, Inc.	74.00	108.00
TRICARE	36.00	68.00

PATIENT INFORMATION FORM

THIS SECTION REFERS TO PATIENT ONLY

Name: Jorge Z. Martinez	Sex: M	Marital Status: ☐ S ☒ M ☐ D ☐ W	Birth Date: 9/16/42

Address: 900 Andover Circle	SS#: 198-22-8463

City: Fairview	State: OH	Zip: 43773	Employer: COSTINC (full-time)	Phone:

Home Phone: 999-555-4009	Employer's Address: 3504 Overland Avenue

Work Phone: 999-555-4300	City: Columbus	State: OH	Zip: 43214

Spouse's Name: Janis Martinez	Spouse's Employer: Computer Consultants

Emergency Contact: Janis Martinez	Relationship: wife	Phone #: 999-555-4009

FILL IN IF PATIENT IS A MINOR

Parent/Guardian's Name:	Sex:	Marital Status: ☐ S ☐ M ☐ D ☐ W	Birth Date:

Phone:	SS#:

Address:	Employer:	Phone:

City:	State:	Zip:	Employer's Address:

Student Status:	City:	State:	Zip:

INSURANCE INFORMATION

Primary Insurance Company: Aetna Health Plans	Secondary Insurance Company:

Subscriber's Name: Jorge Martinez	Birth Date: 9/16/42	Subscriber's Name: Birth Date:

Plan: HMO	SS#: 198-22-8463	Plan:

Policy #: 777JM	Group #: COS-41	Policy #: Group #:

Copayment/Deductible: $15 copay	Price Code: A

OTHER INFORMATION

Reason for visit: burning upon urination	Allergy to Medication (list):

Name of referring physician:	If auto accident, list date and state in which it occurred:

I authorize treatment and agree to pay all fees and charges for the person named above. I agree to pay all charges shown by statements, promptly upon their presentation, unless credit arrangements are agreed upon in writing.

I authorize payment directly to POLARIS MEDICAL GROUP of insurance benefits otherwise payable to me. I hereby authorize the release of any medical information necessary in order to process a claim for payment in my behalf.

Jorge Martinez	6/24/10
(Patient's Signature/Parent or Guardian's Signature)	(Date)

I plan to make payment of my medical expenses as follows (check one or more):

__X__ Insurance (as above)   __X__ Cash/Check/Credit/Debit Card   _____ Medicare   _____ Medicaid   _____ Workers' Comp.

ENCOUNTER FORM

6/24/2010 **4:00pm**	**Dr. Michael Mahabir**
DATE TIME	PROVIDER
Jorge Z. Martinez	**MARTIJO0**
PATIENT NAME	CHART #

OFFICE VISITS - SYMPTOMATIC - NEW		
99201	OF--New Patient Minimal	
99202	OF--New Patient Low	
99203	OF--New Patient Detailed	X
99204	OF--New Patient Moderate	
99205	OF--New Patient High	
OFFICE VISITS - SYMPTOMATIC - ESTABLISHED		
99211	OF--Established Patient Minimal	
99212	OF--Established Patient Low	
99213	OF--Established Patient Detailed	
99214	OF--Established Patient Moderate	
99215	OF--Established Patient High	
PREVENTIVE VISITS - NEW		
99381	Under 1 Year	
99382	1 - 4 Years	
99383	5 - 11 Years	
99384	12 - 17 Years	
99385	18 - 39 Years	
99386	40 - 64 Years	
99387	65 Years & Up	
PREVENTIVE VISITS - ESTABLISHED		
99391	Under 1 Year	
99392	1 - 4 Years	
99393	5 - 11 Years	
99394	12 - 17 Years	
99395	18 - 39 Years	
99396	40 - 64 Years	
99397	65 Years & Up	
HOSPITAL/NURSING HOME VISITS		
99221	Initial hospital care, det.	
99222	Initial hospital care, comp.	
99223	Initial hospital care, high	
99281	ER Visit, min.	
99282	ER Visit, low	
99283	ER Visit, det.	
99284	ER Visit, moderate	
99285	ER Visit, high	
99307	Subseq. nursing facility care, pf.	

PROCEDURES		
10060	Incision/drainage, abcess	
20610	Aspiration, bursa	
29505	Splint, long leg	
29515	Splint, short leg	
36415	Routine venipuncture	
45330	Sigmoidoscopy, flex	
46600	Anoscopy, diagnostic	
71030	Chest x-ray, complete	
73610	Radiology, ankle, complete	
93000	Routine ECG	
93018	Cardiovascular stress test	
99070	Supplies and materials	
LABORATORY		
80050	General health panel	
81000	Urinalysis, complete	X
82270	Blood, occult, feces screening	
82607	Vitamin B-12 test	
82948	Glucose, blood reagent	
85027	CBC, automated	
85651	Sedimentation rate test, manual	
86360	Absolute CD4/CD8 ratio	
86592	Syphilis test	
87070	Throat culture	
87088	Urine culture	X
88150	Cytopathology, cervical or vaginal	
INJECTIONS		
90471	Immunization administration	
90472	Immunization administration, 2nd	
90658	Influenza injection, ages >3	
90702	DT immunization, ages <7	
90703	Tetanus immunization	
90707	MMR immunization	
90722	Therapeutic injection	
90723	DtaP - HepB - IPV	
90732	Pneumococcal immunization	

POLARIS MEDICAL GROUP		NOTES
REFERRING PHYSICIAN	NPI	
AUTHORIZATION #		
DIAGNOSIS 599.0		
PAYMENT AMOUNT $15.00 copay, check #1819		

ENCOUNTER FORM

6/24/2010   **4:30pm**
DATE   TIME

Dr. Robin Crebore
PROVIDER

Susan R. Jonas
PATIENT NAME

JONASSU0
CHART #

OFFICE VISITS - SYMPTOMATIC - NEW		
99201	OF--New Patient Minimal	
99202	OF--New Patient Low	
99203	OF--New Patient Detailed	
99204	OF--New Patient Moderate	
99205	OF--New Patient High	
OFFICE VISITS - SYMPTOMATIC - ESTABLISHED		
99211	OF--Established Patient Minimal	
99212	OF--Established Patient Low	X
99213	OF--Established Patient Detailed	
99214	OF--Established Patient Moderate	
99215	OF--Established Patient High	
PREVENTIVE VISITS - NEW		
99381	Under 1 Year	
99382	1 - 4 Years	
99383	5 - 11 Years	
99384	12 - 17 Years	
99385	18 - 39 Years	
99386	40 - 64 Years	
99387	65 Years & Up	
PREVENTIVE VISITS - ESTABLISHED		
99391	Under 1 Year	
99392	1 - 4 Years	
99393	5 - 11 Years	
99394	12 - 17 Years	
99395	18 - 39 Years	
99396	40 - 64 Years	
99397	65 Years & Up	
HOSPITAL/NURSING HOME VISITS		
99221	Initial hospital care, det.	
99222	Initial hospital care, comp.	
99223	Initial hospital care, high	
99281	ER Visit, min.	
99282	ER Visit, low	
99283	ER Visit, det.	
99284	ER Visit, moderate	
99285	ER Visit, high	
99307	Subseq. nursing facility care, pf.	

PROCEDURES		
10060	Incision/drainage, abcess	
20610	Aspiration, bursa	
29505	Splint, long leg	
29515	Splint, short leg	
36415	Routine venipuncture	
45330	Sigmoidoscopy, flex	
46600	Anoscopy, diagnostic	
71030	Chest x-ray, complete	
73610	Radiology, ankle, complete	
93000	Routine ECG	
93018	Cardiovascular stress test	
99070	Supplies and materials	
LABORATORY		
80050	General health panel	
81000	Urinalysis, complete	
82270	Blood, occult, feces screening	
82607	Vitamin B-12 test	
82948	Glucose, blood reagent	
85027	CBC, automated	
85651	Sedimentation rate test, manual	
86360	Absolute CD4/CD8 ratio	
86592	Syphilis test	
87070	Throat culture	
87088	Urine culture	
88150	Cytopathology, cervical or vaginal	
INJECTIONS		
90471	Immunization administration	
90472	Immunization administration, 2nd	
90658	Influenza injection, ages >3	
90702	DT immunization, ages <7	
90703	Tetanus immunization	
90707	MMR immunization	
90722	Therapeutic injection	
90723	DtaP - HepB - IPV	
90732	Pneumococcal immunization	

POLARIS MEDICAL GROUP

		NOTES
REFERRING PHYSICIAN	NPI	
AUTHORIZATION #		
DIAGNOSIS		
PAYMENT AMOUNT **$15.00 copay, check #349**		

Polaris Medical Group

Name: Susan R. Jonas   **Telephone:** 614-555-9908

Date of Birth: 4/4/71   **Age:** 39

6/24/10   **PROBLEM 1:**   Dermatitis, contact, NOS
                 CHIEF COMPLAINT: Rash

     S: Rash on leg, itching; reports probable exposure to poison ivy.
     O: Swelling, blistering, some scaling of area.
     A: Contact dermatitis, mild.
     P: Topical application of Benadryl® cream.

                 Robin Crebore, M.D.

ENCOUNTER FORM

6/25/2010	9:15am		Dr. Robin Crebore
DATE	TIME		PROVIDER

Martin G. Szinovacz		SZINOMA0
PATIENT NAME		CHART #

OFFICE VISITS - SYMPTOMATIC - NEW		
99201	OF--New Patient Minimal	
99202	OF--New Patient Low	
99203	OF--New Patient Detailed	
99204	OF--New Patient Moderate	
99205	OF--New Patient High	

OFFICE VISITS - SYMPTOMATIC - ESTABLISHED		
99211	OF--Established Patient Minimal	
99212	OF--Established Patient Low	
99213	OF--Established Patient Detailed	X
99214	OF--Established Patient Moderate	
99215	OF--Established Patient High	

PREVENTIVE VISITS - NEW		
99381	Under 1 Year	
99382	1 - 4 Years	
99383	5 - 11 Years	
99384	12 - 17 Years	
99385	18 - 39 Years	
99386	40 - 64 Years	
99387	65 Years & Up	

PREVENTIVE VISITS - ESTABLISHED		
99391	Under 1 Year	
99392	1 - 4 Years	
99393	5 - 11 Years	
99394	12 - 17 Years	
99395	18 - 39 Years	
99396	40 - 64 Years	
99397	65 Years & Up	

HOSPITAL/NURSING HOME VISITS		
99221	Initial hospital care, det.	
99222	Initial hospital care, comp.	
99223	Initial hospital care, high	
99281	ER Visit, min.	
99282	ER Visit, low	
99283	ER Visit, det.	
99284	ER Visit, moderate	
99285	ER Visit, high	
99307	Subseq. nursing facility care, pf.	

PROCEDURES		
10060	Incision/drainage, abcess	
20610	Aspiration, bursa	
29505	Splint, long leg	
29515	Splint, short leg	
36415	Routine venipuncture	
45330	Sigmoidoscopy, flex	
46600	Anoscopy, diagnostic	
71030	Chest x-ray, complete	
73610	Radiology, ankle, complete	
93000	Routine ECG	
93018	Cardiovascular stress test	
99070	Supplies and materials	

LABORATORY		
80050	General health panel	
81000	Urinalysis, complete	
82270	Blood, occult, feces screening	
82607	Vitamin B-12 test	
82948	Glucose, blood reagent	
85027	CBC, automated	
85651	Sedimentation rate test, manual	
86360	Absolute CD4/CD8 ratio	
86592	Syphilis test	
87070	Throat culture	
87088	Urine culture	
88150	Cytopathology, cervical or vaginal	

INJECTIONS		
90471	Immunization administration	
90472	Immunization administration, 2nd	
90658	Influenza injection, ages >3	
90702	DT immunization, ages <7	
90703	Tetanus immunization	
90707	MMR immunization	
90722	Therapeutic injection	
90723	DtaP - HepB - IPV	
90732	Pneumococcal immunization	

POLARIS MEDICAL GROUP		NOTES
REFERRING PHYSICIAN	NPI	
AUTHORIZATION #		
DIAGNOSIS 401.1		
PAYMENT AMOUNT $15.00 copay, check #3404		

PATIENT INFORMATION FORM

THIS SECTION REFERS TO PATIENT ONLY

Name: Eugene S. Kadar			Sex: M	Marital Status: ☒ S ☐ M ☐ D ☐ W	Birth Date: 6/1/77

Address: 8003 Oxford Lane			SS#: 499-09-7453		

City: Highland	State: OH	Zip: 45132	Employer: Columbus Insurance Company (full-time)		Phone:

Home Phone: 999-555-5858	Employer's Address: 9800 Overland Avenue

Work Phone: 999-555-1212	City: Columbus	State: OH	Zip: 43214

Spouse's Name:	Spouse's Employer:

Emergency Contact: Roger Kadar	Relationship: brother	Phone #: 999-555-4443

FILL IN IF PATIENT IS A MINOR

Parent/Guardian's Name:	Sex:	Marital Status: ☐ S ☐ M ☐ D ☐ W	Birth Date:

Phone:	SS#:

Address:	Employer:	Phone:

City:	State:	Zip:	Employer's Address:

Student Status:	City:	State:	Zip:

INSURANCE INFORMATION

Primary Insurance Company: Cigna Healthplan	Secondary Insurance Company:

Subscriber's Name: Eugene Kadar	Birth Date: 6/1/77	Subscriber's Name:	Birth Date:

Plan: HMO	SS#: 499-09-7453	Plan:

Policy #: 762-TTY	Group #: BBA998534	Policy #:	Group #:

Copayment/Deductible: $18 copay	Price Code: A	

OTHER INFORMATION

Reason for visit: sores on lip	Allergy to Medication (list):

Name of referring physician:	If auto accident, list date and state in which it occurred:

I authorize treatment and agree to pay all fees and charges for the person named above. I agree to pay all charges shown by statements, promptly upon their presentation, unless credit arrangements are agreed upon in writing.

I authorize payment directly to POLARIS MEDICAL GROUP of insurance benefits otherwise payable to me. I hereby authorize the release of any medical information necessary in order to process a claim for payment in my behalf.

Eugene S. Kadar   6/25/10

(Patient's Signature/Parent or Guardian's Signature)   (Date)

I plan to make payment of my medical expenses as follows (check one or more):

_X_ Insurance (as above)   _X_ Cash/Check/Credit/Debit Card   ___ Medicare   ___ Medicaid   ___ Workers' Comp.

ENCOUNTER FORM

6/25/2010 10:15am	Dr. Robin Crebore
DATE TIME	PROVIDER
Eugene S. Kadar	KADAREU0
PATIENT NAME	CHART #

OFFICE VISITS - SYMPTOMATIC - NEW		
99201	OF--New Patient Minimal	
99202	OF--New Patient Low	X
99203	OF--New Patient Detailed	
99204	OF--New Patient Moderate	
99205	OF--New Patient High	
OFFICE VISITS - SYMPTOMATIC - ESTABLISHED		
99211	OF--Established Patient Minimal	
99212	OF--Established Patient Low	
99213	OF--Established Patient Detailed	
99214	OF--Established Patient Moderate	
99215	OF--Established Patient High	
PREVENTIVE VISITS - NEW		
99381	Under 1 Year	
99382	1 - 4 Years	
99383	5 - 11 Years	
99384	12 - 17 Years	
99385	18 - 39 Years	
99386	40 - 64 Years	
99387	65 Years & Up	
PREVENTIVE VISITS - ESTABLISHED		
99391	Under 1 Year	
99392	1 - 4 Years	
99393	5 - 11 Years	
99394	12 - 17 Years	
99395	18 - 39 Years	
99396	40 - 64 Years	
99397	65 Years & Up	
HOSPITAL/NURSING HOME VISITS		
99221	Initial hospital care, det.	
99222	Initial hospital care, comp.	
99223	Initial hospital care, high	
99281	ER Visit, min.	
99282	ER Visit, low	
99283	ER Visit, det.	
99284	ER Visit, moderate	
99285	ER Visit, high	
99307	Subseq. nursing facility care, pf.	

PROCEDURES		
10060	Incision/drainage, abcess	
20610	Aspiration, bursa	
29505	Splint, long leg	
29515	Splint, short leg	
36415	Routine venipuncture	
45330	Sigmoidoscopy, flex	
46600	Anoscopy, diagnostic	
71030	Chest x-ray, complete	
73610	Radiology, ankle, complete	
93000	Routine ECG	
93018	Cardiovascular stress test	
99070	Supplies and materials	
LABORATORY		
80050	General health panel	
81000	Urinalysis, complete	
82270	Blood, occult, feces screening	
82607	Vitamin B-12 test	
82948	Glucose, blood reagent	
85027	CBC, automated	
85651	Sedimentation rate test, manual	
86360	Absolute CD4/CD8 ratio	
86592	Syphilis test	
87070	Throat culture	
87088	Urine culture	
88150	Cytopathology, cervical or vaginal	
INJECTIONS		
90471	Immunization administration	
90472	Immunization administration, 2nd	
90658	Influenza injection, ages >3	
90702	DT immunization, ages <7	
90703	Tetanus immunization	
90707	MMR immunization	
90722	Therapeutic injection	
90723	DtaP - HepB - IPV	
90732	Pneumococcal immunization	

POLARIS MEDICAL GROUP

		NOTES
REFERRING PHYSICIAN	NPI	
AUTHORIZATION #		
DIAGNOSIS herpes simplex		
PAYMENT AMOUNT $18.00 copay, check #2039		

PATIENT INFORMATION FORM

THIS SECTION REFERS TO PATIENT ONLY

Name: William R. Nisinson	Sex: M	Marital Status: ☐ S ☐ M ☒ D ☐ W	Birth Date: 6/12/64

Address:
459 Radford Street

SS#:
336-97-9162

City: Homeworth	State: OH	Zip: 43909	Employer: Dan's Hardware (full-time)	Phone:

Home Phone:
999-555-5757

Employer's Address:
3778 Old Turnpike

Work Phone: 999-555-3200	City: Cincinnati	State: OH	Zip: 43999

Spouse's Name:

Spouse's Employer:

Emergency Contact: John Nisinson	Relationship: brother	Phone #: 999-555-0321

FILL IN IF PATIENT IS A MINOR

Parent/Guardian's Name:	Sex:	Marital Status: ☐ S ☐ M ☐ D ☐ W	Birth Date:

Phone:

SS#:

Address:

Employer: Phone:

City:	State:	Zip:	Employer's Address:

Student Status:	City:	State:	Zip:

INSURANCE INFORMATION

Primary Insurance Company:

Workers' Compensation - BCBS of Ohio

Secondary Insurance Company:

Subscriber's Name:	Birth Date:	Subscriber's Name:	Birth Date:

Plan:	SS#:	Plan:

Policy #:	Group #:	Policy #:	Group #:

Copayment/Deductible:	Price Code: A	

OTHER INFORMATION

Reason for visit: fall while on the job (WC)	Allergy to Medication (list):

Name of referring physician:	If auto accident, list date and state in which it occurred:

I authorize treatment and agree to pay all fees and charges for the person named above. I agree to pay all charges shown by statements, promptly upon their presentation, unless credit arrangements are agreed upon in writing.

I authorize payment directly to POLARIS MEDICAL GROUP of insurance benefits otherwise payable to me. I hereby authorize the release of any medical information necessary in order to process a claim for payment in my behalf.

William R. Nisinson   6/25/10

(Patient's Signature/Parent or Guardian's Signature)   (Date)

I plan to make payment of my medical expenses as follows (check one or more):

_____ Insurance (as above)   _____ Cash/Check/Credit/Debit Card   _____ Medicare   _____ Medicaid   _X_ Workers' Comp.

ENCOUNTER FORM

6/25/2010   12:00pm   Dr. Michael Mahabir
DATE   TIME   PROVIDER

William R. Nisinson   NISINWI0
PATIENT NAME   CHART #

OFFICE VISITS - SYMPTOMATIC - NEW		
99201	OF--New Patient Minimal	
99202	OF--New Patient Low	X
99203	OF--New Patient Detailed	
99204	OF--New Patient Moderate	
99205	OF--New Patient High	
OFFICE VISITS - SYMPTOMATIC - ESTABLISHED		
99211	OF--Established Patient Minimal	
99212	OF--Established Patient Low	
99213	OF--Established Patient Detailed	
99214	OF--Established Patient Moderate	
99215	OF--Established Patient High	
PREVENTIVE VISITS - NEW		
99381	Under 1 Year	
99382	1 - 4 Years	
99383	5 - 11 Years	
99384	12 - 17 Years	
99385	18 - 39 Years	
99386	40 - 64 Years	
99387	65 Years & Up	
PREVENTIVE VISITS - ESTABLISHED		
99391	Under 1 Year	
99392	1 - 4 Years	
99393	5 - 11 Years	
99394	12 - 17 Years	
99395	18 - 39 Years	
99396	40 - 64 Years	
99397	65 Years & Up	
HOSPITAL/NURSING HOME VISITS		
99221	Initial hospital care, det.	
99222	Initial hospital care, comp.	
99223	Initial hospital care, high	
99281	ER Visit, min.	
99282	ER Visit, low	
99283	ER Visit, det.	
99284	ER Visit, moderate	
99285	ER Visit, high	
99307	Subseq. nursing facility care, pf.	

PROCEDURES		
10060	Incision/drainage, abcess	
20610	Aspiration, bursa	
29505	Splint, long leg	
29515	Splint, short leg	X
36415	Routine venipuncture	
45330	Sigmoidoscopy, flex	
46600	Anoscopy, diagnostic	
71030	Chest x-ray, complete	
73610	Radiology, ankle, complete	X
93000	Routine ECG	
93018	Cardiovascular stress test	
99070	Supplies and materials	
LABORATORY		
80050	General health panel	
81000	Urinalysis, complete	
82270	Blood, occult, feces screening	
82607	Vitamin B-12 test	
82948	Glucose, blood reagent	
85027	CBC, automated	
85651	Sedimentation rate test, manual	
86360	Absolute CD4/CD8 ratio	
86592	Syphilis test	
87070	Throat culture	
87088	Urine culture	
88150	Cytopathology, cervical or vaginal	
INJECTIONS		
90471	Immunization administration	
90472	Immunization administration, 2nd	
90658	Influenza injection, ages >3	
90702	DT immunization, ages <7	
90703	Tetanus immunization	
90707	MMR immunization	
90722	Therapeutic injection	
90723	DtaP - HepB - IPV	
90732	Pneumococcal immunization	

POLARIS MEDICAL GROUP

NOTES

REFERRING PHYSICIAN   NPI

AUTHORIZATION #

DIAGNOSIS
824.8

PAYMENT AMOUNT

ENCOUNTER FORM

6/25/2010	2:45pm	Dr. Michael Mahabir
DATE	TIME	PROVIDER

Daniel Connolly	CONNODA0
PATIENT NAME	CHART #

OFFICE VISITS - SYMPTOMATIC - NEW		
99201	OF--New Patient Minimal	
99202	OF--New Patient Low	
99203	OF--New Patient Detailed	
99204	OF--New Patient Moderate	
99205	OF--New Patient High	
OFFICE VISITS - SYMPTOMATIC - ESTABLISHED		
99211	OF--Established Patient Minimal	
99212	OF--Established Patient Low	X
99213	OF--Established Patient Detailed	
99214	OF--Established Patient Moderate	
99215	OF--Established Patient High	
PREVENTIVE VISITS - NEW		
99381	Under 1 Year	
99382	1 - 4 Years	
99383	5 - 11 Years	
99384	12 - 17 Years	
99385	18 - 39 Years	
99386	40 - 64 Years	
99387	65 Years & Up	
PREVENTIVE VISITS - ESTABLISHED		
99391	Under 1 Year	
99392	1 - 4 Years	
99393	5 - 11 Years	
99394	12 - 17 Years	
99395	18 - 39 Years	
99396	40 - 64 Years	
99397	65 Years & Up	
HOSPITAL/NURSING HOME VISITS		
99221	Initial hospital care, det.	
99222	Initial hospital care, comp.	
99223	Initial hospital care, high	
99281	ER Visit, min.	
99282	ER Visit, low	
99283	ER Visit, det.	
99284	ER Visit, moderate	
99285	ER Visit, high	
99307	Subseq. nursing facility care, pf.	

PROCEDURES		
10060	Incision/drainage, abcess	
20610	Aspiration, bursa	
29505	Splint, long leg	
29515	Splint, short leg	
36415	Routine venipuncture	
45330	Sigmoidoscopy, flex	
46600	Anoscopy, diagnostic	
71030	Chest x-ray, complete	
73610	Radiology, ankle, complete	
93000	Routine ECG	
93018	Cardiovascular stress test	
99070	Supplies and materials	
LABORATORY		
80050	General health panel	
81000	Urinalysis, complete	
82270	Blood, occult, feces screening	
82607	Vitamin B-12 test	
82948	Glucose, blood reagent	
85027	CBC, automated	
85651	Sedimentation rate test, manual	
86360	Absolute CD4/CD8 ratio	
86592	Syphilis test	
87070	Throat culture	
87088	Urine culture	
88150	Cytopathology, cervical or vaginal	
INJECTIONS		
90471	Immunization administration	
90472	Immunization administration, 2nd	
90658	Influenza injection, ages >3	
90702	DT immunization, ages <7	
90703	Tetanus immunization	
90707	MMR immunization	
90722	Therapeutic injection	
90723	DtaP - HepB - IPV	
90732	Pneumococcal immunization	

POLARIS MEDICAL GROUP		NOTES
REFERRING PHYSICIAN	NPI	
AUTHORIZATION #		
DIAGNOSIS 719.45		
PAYMENT AMOUNT		

Physician's Notes

Patient: Yomo Hirosha

Subject: Hospital Visit, Emergency Dept., 6/25/10

ICD: 414.9

CPT: 99283

PATIENT INFORMATION FORM

THIS SECTION REFERS TO PATIENT ONLY

Name: Marilyn K. Rennagel	Sex: F	Marital Status: ☐ S ☒ M ☐ D ☐ W	Birth Date: 6/12/59

Address: 46 Brossard Avenue	SS#: 445-98-2415	

City: Columbus	State: OH	Zip: 43214	Employer: Columbus World Press (full-time)	Phone:

Home Phone: 999-555-8574	Employer's Address: 2399 Overland Way

Work Phone:	City: Columbus	State: OH	Zip: 43214

Spouse's Name:	Spouse's Employer:

Emergency Contact:	Relationship:	Phone #:

FILL IN IF PATIENT IS A MINOR

Parent/Guardian's Name:	Sex:	Marital Status: ☐ S ☐ M ☐ D ☐ W	Birth Date:

Phone:	SS#:

Address:	Employer:	Phone:

City:	State:	Zip:	Employer's Address:

Student Status:	City:	State:	Zip:

INSURANCE INFORMATION

Primary Insurance Company: Blue Cross Blue Shield of Ohio	Secondary Insurance Company:

Subscriber's Name: Marilyn K. Rennagel	Birth Date: 6/12/59	Subscriber's Name:	Birth Date:

Plan: Standard	SS#: 445-98-2415	Plan:

Policy #: XGS0007613045	Group #: 067544-000	Policy #:	Group #:

Copayment/Deductible: $500 deductible	Price Code: A	

OTHER INFORMATION

Reason for visit: diabetes	Allergy to Medication (list):

Name of referring physician:	If auto accident, list date and state in which it occurred:

I authorize treatment and agree to pay all fees and charges for the person named above. I agree to pay all charges shown by statements, promptly upon their presentation, unless credit arrangements are agreed upon in writing.

I authorize payment directly to POLARIS MEDICAL GROUP of insurance benefits otherwise payable to me. I hereby authorize the release of any medical information necessary in order to process a claim for payment in my behalf.

Marilyn K. Rennagel	6/25/10
(Patient's Signature/Parent or Guardian's Signature)	(Date)

I plan to make payment of my medical expenses as follows (check one or more):

__X__ Insurance (as above) __X__ Cash/Check/Credit/Debit Card _____ Medicare _____ Medicaid _____ Workers' Comp.

ENCOUNTER FORM

6/25/2010	3:00pm		Dr. Robin Crebore
DATE	TIME		PROVIDER
Marilyn K. Rennagel			RENNAMA0
PATIENT NAME			CHART #

OFFICE VISITS - SYMPTOMATIC - NEW		
99201	OF--New Patient Minimal	
99202	OF--New Patient Low	
99203	OF--New Patient Detailed	
99204	OF--New Patient Moderate	
99205	OF--New Patient High	

OFFICE VISITS - SYMPTOMATIC - ESTABLISHED		
99211	OF--Established Patient Minimal	
99212	OF--Established Patient Low	
99213	OF--Established Patient Detailed	X
99214	OF--Established Patient Moderate	
99215	OF--Established Patient High	

PREVENTIVE VISITS - NEW		
99381	Under 1 Year	
99382	1 - 4 Years	
99383	5 - 11 Years	
99384	12 - 17 Years	
99385	18 - 39 Years	
99386	40 - 64 Years	
99387	65 Years & Up	

PREVENTIVE VISITS - ESTABLISHED		
99391	Under 1 Year	
99392	1 - 4 Years	
99393	5 - 11 Years	
99394	12 - 17 Years	
99395	18 - 39 Years	
99396	40 - 64 Years	
99397	65 Years & Up	

HOSPITAL/NURSING HOME VISITS		
99221	Initial hospital care, det.	
99222	Initial hospital care, comp.	
99223	Initial hospital care, high	
99281	ER Visit, min.	
99282	ER Visit, low	
99283	ER Visit, det.	
99284	ER Visit, moderate	
99285	ER Visit, high	
99307	Subseq. nursing facility care, pf.	

PROCEDURES		
10060	Incision/drainage, abcess	
20610	Aspiration, bursa	
29505	Splint, long leg	
29515	Splint, short leg	
36415	Routine venipuncture	
45330	Sigmoidoscopy, flex	
46600	Anoscopy, diagnostic	
71030	Chest x-ray, complete	
73610	Radiology, ankle, complete	
93000	Routine ECG	
93018	Cardiovascular stress test	
99070	Supplies and materials	

LABORATORY		
80050	General health panel	
81000	Urinalysis, complete	X
82270	Blood, occult, feces screening	
82607	Vitamin B-12 test	
82948	Glucose, blood reagent	X
85027	CBC, automated	
85651	Sedimentation rate test, manual	
86360	Absolute CD4/CD8 ratio	
86592	Syphilis test	
87070	Throat culture	
87088	Urine culture	
88150	Cytopathology, cervical or vaginal	

INJECTIONS		
90471	Immunization administration	
90472	Immunization administration, 2nd	
90658	Influenza injection, ages >3	
90702	DT immunization, ages <7	
90703	Tetanus immunization	
90707	MMR immunization	
90722	Therapeutic injection	
90723	DtaP - HepB - IPV	
90732	Pneumococcal immunization	

POLARIS MEDICAL GROUP		NOTES
REFERRING PHYSICIAN	NPI	
AUTHORIZATION #		
DIAGNOSIS		
250.00, 414.00		
PAYMENT AMOUNT		

ENCOUNTER FORM

6/25/2010 3:15pm	Dr. Robin Crebore
DATE TIME	PROVIDER
William A. Brown	BROWNWI0
PATIENT NAME	CHART #

OFFICE VISITS - SYMPTOMATIC - NEW		
99201	OF--New Patient Minimal	
99202	OF--New Patient Low	
99203	OF--New Patient Detailed	
99204	OF--New Patient Moderate	
99205	OF--New Patient High	
OFFICE VISITS - SYMPTOMATIC - ESTABLISHED		
99211	OF--Established Patient Minimal	
99212	OF--Established Patient Low	X
99213	OF--Established Patient Detailed	
99214	OF--Established Patient Moderate	
99215	OF--Established Patient High	
PREVENTIVE VISITS - NEW		
99381	Under 1 Year	
99382	1 - 4 Years	
99383	5 - 11 Years	
99384	12 - 17 Years	
99385	18 - 39 Years	
99386	40 - 64 Years	
99387	65 Years & Up	
PREVENTIVE VISITS - ESTABLISHED		
99391	Under 1 Year	
99392	1 - 4 Years	
99393	5 - 11 Years	
99394	12 - 17 Years	
99395	18 - 39 Years	
99396	40 - 64 Years	
99397	65 Years & Up	
HOSPITAL/NURSING HOME VISITS		
99221	Initial hospital care, det.	
99222	Initial hospital care, comp.	
99223	Initial hospital care, high	
99281	ER Visit, min.	
99282	ER Visit, low	
99283	ER Visit, det.	
99284	ER Visit, moderate	
99285	ER Visit, high	
99307	Subseq. nursing facility care, pf.	

PROCEDURES		
10060	Incision/drainage, abcess	
20610	Aspiration, bursa	
29505	Splint, long leg	
29515	Splint, short leg	
36415	Routine venipuncture	
45330	Sigmoidoscopy, flex	
46600	Anoscopy, diagnostic	
71030	Chest x-ray, complete	
73610	Radiology, ankle, complete	
93000	Routine ECG	
93018	Cardiovascular stress test	
99070	Supplies and materials	
LABORATORY		
80050	General health panel	
81000	Urinalysis, complete	
82270	Blood, occult, feces screening	
82607	Vitamin B-12 test	
82948	Glucose, blood reagent	
85027	CBC, automated	
85651	Sedimentation rate test, manual	
86360	Absolute CD4/CD8 ratio	
86592	Syphilis test	
87070	Throat culture	
87088	Urine culture	
88150	Cytopathology, cervical or vaginal	
INJECTIONS		
90471	Immunization administration	
90472	Immunization administration, 2nd	
90658	Influenza injection, ages >3	
90702	DT immunization, ages <7	
90703	Tetanus immunization	
90707	MMR immunization	
90722	Therapeutic injection	
90723	DtaP - HepB - IPV	
90732	Pneumococcal immunization	

POLARIS MEDICAL GROUP

		NOTES
REFERRING PHYSICIAN	NPI	
AUTHORIZATION #		
DIAGNOSIS		
455.5		
PAYMENT AMOUNT		

Standard Health Care
1500 Summit Avenue, Suite 500
Cincinnati, OH 45000

Polaris Medical Group
2100 Grace Avenue
Columbus, OH 43214

Practice ID: 01-234567

Date Prepared: 6/22/10   EFT Number: 0347914

Patient's Name	Dates of Service From - Thru	POS	Proc	Qty	Charge Amount	Allowed Amount	Patient Resp.	Amt. Paid Provider
Daiute, Angelo X	6/17/10 - 6/17/10	11	99386	1	$233.00	$180.00	$15.00	$165.00
Daiute, Angelo X	6/17/10 - 6/17/10	11	36415	1	$22.00	$17.00	$0.00	$17.00
Daiute, Angelo X	6/17/10 - 6/17/10	11	93000	1	$84.00	$70.00	$0.00	$70.00
Daiute, Angelo X	6/17/10 - 6/17/10	11	80050	1	$143.00	$120.00	$0.00	$120.00
Daiute, Angelo X	6/17/10 - 6/17/10	11	81000	1	$22.00	$17.00	$0.00	$17.00
Totals					$504.00	$404.00	$15.00	$389.00

* * * * * * * *   *EFT transmitted in the amount of $389.00*   * * * * * * * *

Ohio Insurance Company
1600 Galleria Way
Cleveland, OH 44000

Polaris Medical Group
2100 Grace Avenue
Columbus, OH 43214

Practice ID: 09-012345

Date Prepared: 6/30/10   EFT Number: 115896

Patient's Name	Dates of Service From - Thru	POS	Proc	Qty	Charge Amount	Allowed Amount	Patient Resp.	Amt. Paid Provider
Ferrara, Victoria	6/16/10 - 6/16/10	11	99212	1	$54.00	$54.00	$5.40	$48.60
Totals					$54.00	$54.00	$5.40	$48.60

* * * * * * * *   *EFT transmitted in the amount of $48.60*   * * * * * * * *

Standard Health Care
1500 Summit Avenue, Suite 500
Cincinnati, OH 45000

Polaris Medical Group
2100 Grace Avenue
Columbus, OH 43214

Practice ID: 01-234567

Date Prepared: 6/30/10   EFT Number: 65891372

Patient's Name	Dates of Service From - Thru	POS	Proc	Qty	Charge Amount	Allowed Amount	Patient Resp.	Amt. Paid Provider
Kavanaugh, Gregory	6/14/10 - 6/14/10	11	99212	1	$54.00	$46.00	$15.00	$31.00
Kavanaugh, Gregory	6/14/10 - 6/14/10	11	36415	1	$22.00	$17.00	$0.00	$17.00
Kavanaugh, Gregory	6/14/10 - 6/14/10	11	86360	1	$263.00	$195.00	$0.00	$195.00
Szinovacz, Martin G	6/25/10 - 6/25/10	11	99213	1	$72.00	$62.00	$15.00	$47.00
Totals					$411.00	$320.00	$30.00	$290.00

* * * * * * * *   *EFT transmitted in the amount of $290.00*   * * * * * * * *

Blue Cross Blue Shield of Ohio
5000 First Street
Worthington, OH 43085

Polaris Medical Group
2100 Grace Avenue
Columbus, OH 43214

Practice ID: 04-5678901

Date Prepared: 6/30/10   EFT Number: 9928674

Patient's Name	Dates of Service From - Thru	POS	Proc	Qty	Charge Amount	Allowed Amount	Patient Resp.	Amt. Paid Provider
Berkel-Rees, Gloria	6/18/10 - 6/18/10	11	99213	1	$72.00	$72.00	$21.60	$50.40
Berkel-Rees, Gloria	6/18/10 - 6/18/10	11	99070	1	$15.00	$15.00	$4.50	$10.50
Brown, William A	6/15/10 - 6/15/10	11	99214	1	$105.00	$105.00	$31.50	$73.50
Brown, William A	6/15/10 - 6/15/10	11	82270	1	$19.00	$19.00	$5.70	$13.30
Brown, William A	6/15/10 - 6/15/10	11	46600	1	$89.00	$89.00	$26.70	$62.30
Brown, William A	6/25/10 - 6/25/10	11	99212	1	$54.00	$54.00	$16.20	$37.80
Ferrone, Fran C	6/21/10 - 6/21/10	11	99202	1	$88.00	$88.00	$26.40	$61.60
LeConey, James I	6/15/10 - 6/15/10	11	99214	1	$105.00	$105.00	$31.50	$73.50
O'Keefe, Diana E	6/22/10 - 6/22/10	11	99211	1	$36.00	$36.00	$10.80	$25.20
O'Keefe, Diana E	6/22/10 - 6/22/10	11	85651	1	$24.00	$24.00	$7.20	$16.80
Rennagel, Marilyn K	6/25/10 - 6/25/10	11	99213	1	$72.00	$72.00	$21.60	$50.40
Rennagel, Marilyn K	6/25/10 - 6/25/10	11	81000	1	$22.00	$22.00	$6.60	$15.40
Rennagel, Marilyn K	6/25/10 - 6/25/10	11	82948	1	$18.00	$18.00	$5.40	$12.60

| Totals | | | | | $719.00 | $719.00 | $215.70 | $503.30 |

* * * * * * *   *EFT transmitted in the amount of $503.30*   * * * * * * *

Blue Cross Blue Shield of Ohio - Workers' Compensation
5000 First Street
Worthington, OH 43085

Polaris Medical Group
2100 Grace Avenue
Columbus, OH 43214

Practice ID: 02-3456789

Date Prepared: 6/30/10   EFT Number: 88415629

Patient's Name	Dates of Service From - Thru	POS	Proc	Qty	Charge Amount	Allowed Amount	Patient Resp.	Amt. Paid Provider
Nisinson, William R	6/25/10 - 6/25/10	11	99202	1	$88.00	$88.00	$0.00	$88.00
Nisinson, William R	6/25/10 - 6/25/10	11	29515	1	$114.00	$114.00	$0.00	$114.00
Nisinson, William R	6/25/10 - 6/25/10	11	73610	1	$113.00	$113.00	$0.00	$113.00
Totals					$315.00	$315.00	$0.00	$315.00

* * * * * * * *   *EFT transmitted in the amount of $315.00*   * * * * * * * *

Nationwide Medicare HMO
P.O. Box 7000
Columbus, OH 43214

Polaris Medical Group
2100 Grace Avenue
Columbus, OH 43214

Practice ID: 10-123456

Date Prepared: 6/30/10   EFT Number: 378214

Patient's Name	Dates of Service From - Thru	POS	Proc	Qty	Charge Amount	Allowed Amount	Patient Resp.	Amt. Paid Provider
Atchely, Rachel D	5/26/10 - 5/26/10	31	99311	1	$63.00	$34.00	$5.00	$29.00
Atchely, Rachel D	6/23/10 - 6/23/10	31	99311	1	$63.00	$34.00	$5.00	$29.00
Beedon, Myrna E	5/31/10 - 5/31/10	11	99211	1	$36.00	$14.00	$5.00	$9.00
Beedon, Myrna E	5/31/10 - 5/31/10	11	93000	1	$84.00	$29.00	$0.00	$29.00
Beedon, Myrna E	6/21/10 - 6/21/10	21	99222	1	$205.00	$113.00	$0.00	$113.00
Estephan, Wilma T	6/15/10 - 6/15/10	11	99202	1	$88.00	$50.00	$5.00	$45.00
Estephan, Wilma T	6/15/10 - 6/15/10	11	81000	1	$22.00	$10.00	$0.00	$10.00
Estephan, Wilma T	6/15/10 - 6/15/10	11	87088	1	$42.00	$18.00	$0.00	$18.00
McAniff, Nora B	6/16/10 - 6/16/10	11	99202	1	$88.00	$50.00	$5.00	$45.00
Torres-Gil, Flora K	6/22/10 - 6/22/10	11	20610	1	$112.00	$45.00	$5.00	$40.00
Wong, Hanna Z	6/24/10 - 6/24/10	11	99205	1	$229.00	$128.00	$5.00	$123.00
Wong, Hanna Z	6/24/10 - 6/24/10	11	93000	1	$84.00	$29.00	$0.00	$29.00
Totals					$1116.00	$554.00	$35.00	$519.00

* * * * * * * *   *EFT transmitted in the amount of $519.00*   * * * * * * * *

TRICARE
PO Box 1000
Columbus, OH 43214

Polaris Medical Group
2100 Grace Avenue
Columbus, OH 43214

Practice ID: 05-678901

Date Prepared: 6/30/10 EFT Number: 69876542

Patient's Name	Dates of Service From - Thru	POS	Proc	Qty	Charge Amount	Allowed Amount	Patient Resp.	Amt. Paid Provider
Kopelman, Mary A.	6/14/10 - 6/14/10	11	99202	1	$88.00	$50.00	$10.00	$40.00
Kopelman, Mary A.	6/14/10 - 6/14/10	11	80050	1	$143.00	$70.00	$0.00	$70.00
Kopelman, Mary A.	6/14/10 - 6/14/10	11	36415	1	$22.00	$8.00	$0.00	$8.00
Wu, Elizabeth I	6/21/10 - 6/21/10	11	99212	1	$54.00	$28.00	$10.00	$18.00
Totals					$307.00	$156.00	$20.00	$136.00

* * * * * * * *   *EFT transmitted in the amount of $136.00*   * * * * * * * *

Nationwide Medicare
P.O. Box 7001
Columbus, OH 43214

Polaris Medical Group
2100 Grace Avenue
Columbus, OH 43214

Practice ID: 10-123456

Date Prepared: 6/30/10   EFT Number: 3642988

Patient's Name	Dates of Service From - Thru	POS	Proc	Qty	Charge Amount	Allowed Amount	Patient Resp.	Amt. Paid Provider
Ahmadian, George	5/26/10 - 5/26/10	11	99213	1	$72.00	$39.00	$7.80	$31.20
Ahmadian, George	6/17/10 - 6/17/10	11	99215	1	$163.00	$94.00	$18.80	$75.20
Connolly, Daniel	6/03/10 - 6/03/10	11	99397	1	$155.00	118.00	B	$0.00
Connolly, Daniel	6/06/10 - 6/06/10	11	80050	1	$143.00	70.00	B	$0.00
Connolly, Daniel	6/14/10 - 6/14/10	11	99214	1	$105.00	$59.00	B	$47.20
Connolly, Daniel	6/25/10 - 6/25/10	11	99212	1	$54.00	$28.00	B	$22.40
Stephanos, Lydia	6/14/10 - 6/14/10	11	99213	1	$72.00	$39.00	$7.80	$31.20
Stephanos, Lydia	6/14/10 - 6/14/10	11	10060	1	$117.00	$57.00	$11.40	$45.60

B Claim submitted to secondary payer.

| Totals | | | | | $881.00 | $504.00 | $45.80 | $252.80 |

* * * * * * * *   *EFT transmitted in the amount of $252.80*   * * * * * * * *

Ohio Dept. of Human Resources - Medicaid
PO Box 4000
Columbus OH 43214

Polaris Medical Group
2100 Grace Avenue
Columbus, OH 43214

Practice ID: 11-123456

Date Prepared: 6/30/10   EFT Number: 3968452

Patient's Name	Dates of Service From - Thru	POS	Proc	Qty	Charge Amount	Allowed Amount	Patient Resp.	Amt. Paid Provider
Colbs, Seymour	6/18/10 – 6/18/10	11	99213	1	$72.00	$39.00	$8.25	$30.75
Connolly, Daniel	6/14/10 – 6/14/10	11	99214	1	$105.00	$59.00A	$0.00	$11.80
Connolly, Daniel	6/25/10 – 6/25/10	11	99212	1	$ 54.00	$28.00A	$0.00	$5.60
Hellery, Jimmy	5/28/10 – 5/28/10	11	99211	1	$36.00	$14.00	$8.25	$5.75
Hellery, Jimmy	6/21/10 – 6/21/10	11	99212	1	$54.00	$28.00	$8.25	$19.75
Hellery, Jimmy	6/21/10 – 6/21/10	11	87070	1	$48.00	$20.00	$0.00	$20.00
Yange-Sang, Roberta	6/18/10 – 6/18/10	11	99212	1	$54.00	$28.00	$8.25	$19.75

A - Claim forwarded from primary payer.

Totals		$423.00	$216.00	$33.00	$113.40

* * * * * * *   *EFT transmitted in the amount of $113.40*   * * * * * * *

Columbus Medical Care
3000 Arkady Street
Columbus OH 43214

Polaris Medical Group
2100 Grace Avenue
Columbus, OH 43214

Practice ID: 06-789012

Date Prepared: 6/30/10

EFT Number: 00679522

Patient's Name	Dates of Service From - Thru	POS	Proc	Qty	Charge Amount	Allowed Amount	Patient Resp.	Amt. Paid Provider
Deysenrothe, Floyd	6/21/10 – 6/21/10	11	90471	1	$18.00	$14.00	$12.00	$2.00
Deysenrothe, Floyd	6/21/10 – 6/21/10	11	90703	1	$29.00	$24.00	$0.00	$24.00
Deysenrothe, Mae J	6/23/10 – 6/23/10	11	99395	1	$178.00	$137.00	$12.00	$125.00
Deysenrothe, Mae J	6/23/10 – 6/23/10	11	80050	1	$143.00	$120.00	$0.00	$120.00
Deysenrothe, Mae J	6/23/10 – 6/23/10	11	81000	1	$22.00	$17.00	$0.00	$17.00
Deysenrothe, Mae J	6/23/10 – 6/23/10	11	88150	1	$35.00	$29.00	$0.00	$29.00
Deysenrothe, Mae J	6/23/10 – 6/23/10	11	36415	1	$22.00	$17.00	$0.00	$17.00
Deysenrothe, Mae J	6/23/10 – 6/23/10	11	93000	1	$84.00	$70.00	$0.00	$70.00
Deysenrothe, Roger	5/03/10 – 5/03/10	11	99395	1	$178.00	$137.00	$12.00	$125.00
Deysenrothe, Roger	5/03/10 – 5/03/10	11	36415	1	$22.00	$17.00	$0.00	$17.00
Deysenrothe, Roger	5/03/10 – 5/03/10	11	80050	1	$143.00	$120.00	$0.00	$120.00
Deysenrothe, Roger	5/03/10 – 5/03/10	11	81000	1	$22.00	$17.00	$0.00	$17.00
Deysenrothe, Roger	5/03/10 – 5/03/10	11	93000	1	$84.00	$70.00	$0.00	$70.00
Hirosha, Yomo C	4/15/10 – 4/15/10	11	99214	1	$105.00	$91.00	$12.00	$79.00
Hirosha, Yomo C	4/15/10 – 4/15/10	11	93000	1	$84.00	$70.00	$0.00	$70.00
Hirosha, Yomo C	4/15/10 – 4/15/10	11	93018	1	$202.00	$162.00	$0.00	$162.00
Hirosha, Yomo C	6/25/10 – 6/25/10	23	99283	1	$150.00	$131.00	$0.00	$131.00
Weintraub, Stewart	6/16/10 – 6/16/10	23	99283	1	$150.00	$131.00	$0.00	$131.00

| Totals | | | | | $1671.00 | $1374.00 | $48.00 | $1326.00 |

* * * * * * * *   *EFT transmitted in the amount of $1326.00*   * * * * * * * *

Aetna Health Plans
5777 Royal Boulevard
Columbus, OH 43214

Polaris Medical Group
2100 Grace Avenue
Columbus, OH 43214

Practice ID: 08-901234

Date Prepared: 6/30/10   EFT Number: 00059876521

Capitation payment for May 2010 $1500.00
Dr. Robin Crebore
Dr. Michael Mahabir

Capitation payment for June 2010 $1500.00
Dr. Robin Crebore
Dr. Michael Mahabir

* * * * * * * *   *EFT transmitted in the amount of $3000.00*   * * * * * * * *

CIGNA Healthplan
1200 Green Avenue
Cincinnati, OH 45000

Polaris Medical Group
2100 Grace Avenue
Columbus, OH 43214

Practice ID: 07-890123

Date Prepared: 6/30/10   EFT Number: 794620

Capitation payment for May 2010 $2000.00
Dr. Robin Crebore
Dr. Michael Mahabir

Capitation payment for June 2010 $2000.00
Dr. Robin Crebore
Dr. Michael Mahabir

* * * * * * *   *EFT transmitted in the amount of $4000.00*   * * * * * * *

Glossary

accept assignment A physician's agreement to accept an allowed charge as payment in full.

Acknowledgment of Receipt of Notice of Privacy Practices Under the HIPAA Privacy Rule, medical practices must have a written Notice of Privacy Practices that describes the medical office's practices regarding the use and disclosure of Private Health Information (PHI).

allowed amount/allowed charge The amount an insurance carrier or governmental program covers for each service.

assignment of benefits Authorization by a policyholder that allows an insurance carrier to pay benefits directly to a health care provider.

audit A third-party examination of a physician's accounting records or patient records relating to claims.

audit trail A technical safeguard on a computer that keeps track of who has accessed information and when, which is regularly checked by a manager for errors or irregularities in data entry.

authorized signature form A one-time authorization for payment to be made to a physician for services rendered and for the release of medical information to insurance carriers or medical professionals; also called release of information.

benefits (1) The amount of money an insurance carrier pays for services covered by an insurance policy. (2) Nonmonetary employee compensation, such as a paid vacation.

billing compliance program A set of procedures and policies that helps medical office employees comply with applicable laws and regulations and avoid misconduct.

Blue Cross and Blue Shield Association The national licensing agency of Blue Cross and Blue Shield Plans.

breach of confidentiality A party's disclosing to a third party information that was confidential between two original parties.

breach of contract A party's failure to comply with the terms of a legal contract.

CHAMPUS Now the TRICARE program; formerly the Civilian Health and Medical Program of the Uniformed Services for spouses and children of active-duty service members, military retirees and their families, some former spouses, and survivors of deceased military members.

CHAMPVA The Civilian Health and Medical Program of the Veterans Administration (Department of Veterans Affairs), which shares health care costs for families of veterans with 100 percent service-related disabilities and for the surviving spouses and children of veterans who died from service-related disabilities.

COBRA A federal law requiring employers with 20 or more workers who sponsor a group health benefit plan to continue health insurance plan coverage for up to 18 months for terminated or laid-off employees.

CPT The abbreviation that refers to Physician's Current Procedural Terminology.

capitation A method of insurance reimbursement to physicians based on the number of patients seen rather than the services performed.

case A Medisoft term that refers to a grouping of transactions for visits to a physician's office organized around a condition.

Centers for Medicare and Medicaid Services (CMS) The governmental department that runs Medicare and other governmental health programs (formerly HCFA).

chief complaint (CC) A description of the symptoms or other reasons a patient seeks medical care on a particular visit to a physician.

claim appeal A written request for a review of a payment that the provider feels is inadequate or incorrect.

clearinghouse A centralized service bureau that for a fee offers providers the service of receiving electronic media/paper claims, checking and preparing them for processing, and transmitting them in proper data format to the correct carriers.

coding In medical terminology, the process of assigning numerical codes to diagnoses and treatments.

coinsurance The portion of charges under an indemnity plan that the insured must pay for services, based on insurance coverage and payment of a deductible amount.

consultation The service performed by one physician for the purpose of advising an attending physician about a patient's condition and care.

coordination of benefits A clause in an insurance policy that explains how the policy will pay if more than one insurance policy applies to the claim.

copayment The portion or amount of charges that the insured must pay at the time of services, based on insurance coverage and payment of any deductible amounts.

Dx An abbreviation for a physician's diagnosis.

day sheet In a medical office, a report that summarizes the business day's charges and payments, drawn from all the patient ledgers for the day.

deductible The part of medical charges the insured must pay before insurance payment begins.

default The instruction or value a computer is programmed to use unless other instructions or values are entered.

dependent A person related to a policyholder, such as a spouse or child.

diagnosis A physician's opinion of the nature of a patient's illness or injury.

diagnostic code The number assigned to a physician's diagnosis in the International Classification of Diseases (ICD).

dialog box A computer screen display with which a user interacts by providing instructions or selecting from among options.

documentation The chronological recording of facts and observations about a patient's health status in a logical sequence.

electronic data interchange (EDI) The electronic exchange of health care claims, remittance, and eligibility and claim status inquiries.

electronic health record (EHR) Electronic collection and management of health data.

encounter form The part of a patient's medical record that contains the diagnosis, services, and fees for a patient's visit.

established patient A patient who has seen the physician within the past three years.

excluded illness A condition or circumstance specified in a medical insurance contract as not covered.

explanation of Medicare benefits (EOMB) Remittance advice that explains how payment for a Medicare claim was determined.

family practitioner A physician with a general practice rather than a specialty; also called a general practitioner.

fee-for-service A way of charging patients for medical services based on the service performed.

fee schedule A list of charges for services and procedures performed by a physician.

fixed fee schedule A payment method based on a list of maximum fees allowed for specific services.

fraud The intentional misrepresentation of information to obtain a benefit.

grievance Job-related problem that an employee feels should be corrected.

guardian An adult responsible for the care and custody of a minor. The guardian can make decisions regarding the minor's health, care, and maintenance.

Health Insurance Claim Form (CMS-1500) The universal form approved by the American Medical Association and CMS for use in requesting benefits from medical insurance carriers and government health programs.

health maintenance organization (HMO) A managed care health care system under which patients pay fixed periodic rates and receive medical services from an approved list of health care providers specified in their contract.

HIPAA (Health Insurance Portability and Accountability Act of 1996) A federal law governing many aspects of health care, such as electronic transmission standards and the security of health care records.

HIPAA Electronic Health Care Transactions and Code Sets (TCS) HIPAA standards governing the electronic exchange of health information using standard formats and standard code sets.

HIPAA Privacy Rule Legislation that protects individually identifiable health information.

HIPAA Security Rule Legislation that outlines the administrative, technical, and physical safeguards required to prevent unauthorized access to protected health care information.

ICD code A system of diagnostic codes based on the International Classification of Diseases.

indemnity plan An agreement to reimburse a policyholder for health care costs due to illness or accidents.

informed consent A written document in which the physician notifies the patient of a procedure and the accompanying hazards, complications, alternatives, and risks.

inpatient A person admitted to a hospital who generally stays overnight and incurs the hospital's room and board fees.

insurance carrier A company or agency that offers financial protection as a result of a specified event.

insurance claim form A document filed with an insurance carrier to receive benefits.

insurance log A medical office's list of insurance claim forms that have been filed and/or paid.

insured The policyholder, or subscriber, to a medical insurance policy or plan.

International Classification of Diseases (ICD) A publication known as the ICD that lists diagnostic codes assigned by the World Health Organization and used by the U.S. government, American medical insurance carriers, and others.

internist A physician who specializes in the care of adults.

liable Legally responsible.

libel A harmful, written statement about someone.

malfeasance Wrongdoing or misconduct, often by someone who is legally bound to proper actions.

managed care A way of supervising medical care to be sure patients get services they need in the most appropriate, cost-effective setting.

Medicaid A federal and state assistance program that pays for health care services for people with incomes below the national poverty level.

medical insurance A financial plan that covers the cost of hospital and/or medical care due to illness or injury.

medical necessity Payment criterion of third-party payers that requires medical treatments to be appropriate for a patient's diagnosis and to be provided in accordance with generally accepted standards of medical practice.

medical malpractice The failure to use an acceptable level of professional skill when giving medical services that results in injury or harm to a patient.

medical professional liability policy An insurance policy that covers a medical office's personnel for unintentional errors in the medical treatment of patients.

medical record A file that includes the patient information form, the patient's medical history, record of care, progress notes, insurance correspondence, and other correspondence.

Medicare The federal health insurance program for people aged 65 or older and for those with some disabilities and end-stage renal disease.

Medicare beneficiary A person covered by Medicare.

Medicare carrier A private insurance organization under contract with the federal government to administer Medicare Part B claims.

Medicare Fee Schedule (MFS) A list of the allowed fees that are reimbursable to Medicare participating physicians; based on the RBRVS system.

Medicare Part A The part of the Medicare program that pays for hospitalization, care in a skilled nursing facility, home health care, and hospice care.

Medicare Part B The part of the Medicare program that pays for physician services, outpatient hospital services, durable medical equipment, and other services and supplies.

Medicare-participating agreement A document signed by physicians and other providers of medical services who have agreed to accept assignment on all Medicare claims.

Medigap insurance An insurance plan offered by a federally approved private insurance carrier designed to supplement Medicare coverage.

menu A list of choices appearing on a computer screen for selection by a user.

modem A device that converts electronic data from computers into signals that can be transmitted over telephone lines.

modifier ICD: A nonessential word or phrase that helps to define a diagnostic code; CPT: a number indicating a special circumstance that affects a medical procedure in some way, such as surgery being more difficult than usual for some reason.

multiple modifiers More than a single two-digit code used to augment a procedure code.

National Provider Identifier (NPI) A unique identifier assigned to a health care provider that is used in standard transactions, such as health care claims.

new patient A patient who has not received professional services from a physician within the past three years.

nonavailability statement A form required for preauthorization when a TRICARE member seeks medical services in other than a military facility.

nonparticipating (nonPAR) physician A physician or other health care provider who chooses not to join a particular governmental program or insurance carrier's plan.

outpatient A patient who receives health care in a hospital without admission; the length of stay is generally 23 hours or less.

participating (PAR) physician A physician who participates in a governmental program or an insurance carrier's plan.

patient chart See medical record.

patient information form A form that includes a patient's personal, employment, and insurance company data needed to complete an insurance claim form; also known as a registration form.

patient ledger In a medical office, a record of all charges and payments made to a particular patient's account.

patient day sheet A report that summarizes the business day's charges and payments, organized by patient.

patient update form A form that is used to update information about a patient's personal, employment, and insurance company data.

Physician's Current Procedural Terminology (CPT) A publication of the American Medical Association containing a standardized system of codes for medical procedures and diagnostic services.

place of service (POS) code Code that describes a location where medical services are performed.

policyholder A person who buys an insurance plan; insured.

preauthorization Prior authorization from an insurance carrier that must be received before a procedure is covered; also know as precertification.

preexisting condition An illness or disorder that existed before the insured's medical insurance contract went into effect.

preferred provider organization (PPO) A managed care network of health care providers who agree to perform services for member patients at discounted fees.

premium The amount of money paid to an insurance carrier to buy an insurance plan.

primary care physician The physician in a health maintenance organization who directs all aspects of a patient's care, including routine services, referrals to specialists within the system, and supervision of hospital admissions; also known as a gatekeeper.

primary diagnosis The diagnosis that represents the patient's major health problem for a particular insurance claim.

primary insurance The insurance plan that pays benefits first when a patient is covered by more than one medical insurance plan.

primary payer The insurance plan that pays first when a patient is covered by more than one insurance plan or governmental program.

prior authorization number An identifying code assigned by a governmental program or insurance carrier when preauthorization is granted; also called a preauthorization number.

privileged communication Confidential conversation between physician and patient.

procedure code A code that identifies medical or diagnostic services.

procedure day sheet A report that summarizes the business day's charges and payments, organized by procedure code.

prognosis The physician's prediction of the outcome of a disease or injury and the likelihood of recovery.

protected health information (PHI) Individually identifiable health information that is transmitted or maintained by electronic media, such as over the Internet, by computer modem, or on magnetic tape or compact disc.

provider In medical insurance, a professional member of the health care team, such as a physician, who provides services or supplies to the insured.

real-time claims adjudication (RTCA) Electronic health insurance claim processed at patient check-out; allows practice to know what the patient will owe for the visit.

referral The transfer of patient care from one physician to another.

release of information A statement that authorizes the provider to give the insurance carrier information needed to process an insurance claim.

remittance advice (RA) A document from an insurance carrier that reports claim activity and shows how the amount of benefit was determined.

schedule of benefits A list of benefits for which an insurance policy will pay.

secondary insurance The insurance plan that pays benefits after the primary carrier when a patient is covered by more than one medical insurance plan.

SOAP format The documentation of medical records according to the S (subjective data), O (objective data), A (assessment), and P (plan of treatment).

sponsor The uniformed service member in a family qualified for TRICARE or CHAMPVA.

subscriber A person who is enrolled in a Blue Cross and Blue Shield Plan.

superbill A custom-made form used by physicians to note diagnosis and treatment; also known as an encounter form or charge ticket.

supplemental insurance An insurance plan, such as Medigap, that provides benefits for services that are not normally covered by a primary plan.

third-party liability An obligation of an insurance plan or governmental program to pay all or part of a patient's medical costs.

third-party payer A payer of one entity for another, as an insurance company paying a physician for services received by a patient.

traditional plan See indemnity plan.

transaction In a computerized billing system, a financial exchange, such as a deposit of funds into a provider's bank account.

TRICARE A governmental health program offering managed care to dependents of active-duty service members, military retirees and their families, some former spouses, and survivors of deceased military members; formerly called CHAMPUS.

type of service code A code that describes the kind of service performed.

Universal Precautions Techniques issued by the Centers for Disease Control and Prevention to protect health care workers from infection.

V code A number that identifies factors that influence health status or give a patient a reason to contact a health care facility when there is no clear diagnosis or disease process.

walkout receipt In a medical office, a completed form a patient receives after a visit. The walkout receipt contains the details of the resulting diagnosis, services provided, fees, and payments received and due.

workers' compensation insurance A state or federal plan that covers medical care and other benefits for employees who suffer accidental injury or become ill as a result of employment.

write off To discount a patient's fee in accordance with contractual agreements.

X12-837 Health Care Claim, or **837P** The electronic claim format that is used to bill for a physician's services.

Index